The PCOS Recipe Book

Thrive with polycystic ovary syndrome

MEGAN HALLETT
NUTRITIONAL THERAPIST

hamlyn

First published in Great Britain in 2025 by Hamlyn,
an imprint of Octopus Publishing Group Ltd,
Carmelite House, 50 Victoria Embankment,
London EC4Y 0DZ
www.octopusbooks.co.uk
www.octopusbooksusa.com

An Hachette UK Company
www.hachette.co.uk

The authorized representative in the EEA is
Hachette Ireland, 8 Castlecourt Centre, Dublin 15,
D15 XTP3, Ireland (email: info@hbgi.ie)

Distributed in the US by Hachette Book Group,
1290 Avenue of the Americas, 4th and 5th Floors,
New York, NY 10104

Distributed in Canada by Canadian Manda Group,
664 Annette St., Toronto, Ontario, Canada M6S 2C8

ISBN: 978-0-600-63956-5
eISBN: 978-0-600-63957-2

A CIP catalogue record for this book is available
from the British Library.

Printed and bound in China.

10 9 8 7 6 5 4 3 2 1

Comissioned by: Alice Gawthrop
Publisher: Kate Fox
Editor: Scarlet Furness
Art Director: Jaz Bahra
Designer: Nicky Collings
Production Manager: Caroline Alberti

Standard level spoon measurements are used
in all recipes.
1 tablespoon = one 15 ml spoon
1 teaspoon = one 5 ml spoon

Both imperial and metric measurements have been
given in all recipes. Use one set of measurements
only and not a mixture of both.

Eggs should be medium unless otherwise stated.
The Department of Health advises that eggs should
not be consumed raw. It is prudent for more
vulnerable people such as pregnant and nursing
mothers, the elderly, babies and young children
to avoid uncooked or lightly cooked dishes made
with eggs.

Milk should be full fat unless otherwise stated.

Fresh herbs should be used unless otherwise stated.
If unavailable use dried herbs as an alternative but
halve the quantities stated.

Pepper should be freshly ground black pepper
unless otherwise stated.

This book includes dishes made with nuts and nut
derivatives. It is advisable for those with known
allergic reactions to nuts and nut derivatives and
those who may be potentially vulnerable to these
allergies, such as pregnant and nursing mothers, the
elderly, babies and children, to avoid dishes made
with nuts and nut oils. It is also prudent to check the
labels of pre-prepared ingredients for the possible
inclusion of nut derivatives.

Vegetarians should look for the 'V' symbol on a
cheese to ensure it is made with vegetarian rennet.

Polycystic ovary syndrome is a hormone condition
that affects up to 13 per cent of women worldwide
(World Health Organization, 2025).

Contents

Introduction

Megan Hallett, Nutritional Therapist (mBANT, rCNHC)

What is PCOS?

Polycystic Ovary Syndrome (PCOS) is a common yet complex disorder of the endochrine and metabolic systems that affects how a woman's ovaries work.

The endochrine system produces and releases hormones, which regulate bodily functions such as growth, metabolism, reproduction and mood. The hallmark features of PCOS are excess androgens (sex hormones responsible for 'male' characteristics) in the body, which causes symptoms such as oily skin, acne, excess facial or body hair, and thinning hair or hair loss. Other symptoms can include irregular or missed periods, trouble conceiving, weight gain or difficulty losing weight.

While the exact cause of PCOS is unknown, there are many theories around proposed cause and risk factors which include genetics, environmental toxins and exposure to androgens in the womb, to name a few.

There is no cure, but symptoms can be treated. Eating a healthy, well-balanced diet has been shown to improve some symptoms.

The Role of Insulin in PCOS

A common feature of PCOS is insulin resistance, and this is behind many of the symptoms we now associate with PCOS. Insulin is a hormone that regulates blood sugar levels. If insulin levels have been chronically elevated, cells in the body become less responsive to that insulin's action, meaning the body makes more to compensate.

In PCOS, raised insulin drives excess androgens, but can also present other challenges, such as difficulty losing body fat or maintaining a healthy weight and regulating glucose levels. It can lead to short-term feelings of low energy, and long-term issues and complications, such as heart disease and type 2 diabetes. This is because our cells are unable to take in as much glucose, so more remains in the blood instead of being used by our cells for energy.

Insulin increases androgens by stimulating the ovaries to make more of this group of hormones, which includes testosterone. Insulin can also decrease the activity of a binding protein called sex hormone binding globulin (SHBG), which binds to testosterone to make it inactive. The less SHBG, the more free testosterone roaming around the body.

Both high insulin and excess androgens can inhibit ovulation. These hormones prevent the follicles in the ovaries from fully maturing and releasing an egg, causing them to accumulate as small sacs instead of a single mature egg being released. This is what is seen on ultrasound, and is the 'polycystic' part of PCOS. The 'cysts', however, are actually small, immature follicles rather than functional cysts, which can also occur in women without PCOS.

In normal menstrual cycles, luteinizing hormone (LH) triggers the release of an egg around ovulation. In PCOS, an imbalance in LH:FSH (follicle stimulating hormone) is common, and in some cases is used alongside testosterone as a key component of a diagnosis. Rather than peaking at ovulation, LH can remain high across the whole menstrual cycle in response to high insulin levels, and can further impact androgen levels or prevent ovulation from occurring.

When we don't ovulate, we also don't make a hormone called progesterone. With no ovulation occurring, no cyclical LH pulses and no progesterone being made, the menstrual cycle becomes irregular. What's more, high testosterone also increases insulin resistance. As a result, we are stuck in a bit of a cycle!

Diagnosis

Despite PCOS being common, there is still confusion and controversy surrounding diagnosis. The range and severity of symptoms vary, and diagnostic criteria has changed over time.

The first formal criteria for PCOS came from the National Institutes of Health (NIH) in 1990, and required excess androgen and infrequent ovulation to be present. Polycystic ovaries was not included.

In 2004, something called the Rotterdam Criteria was created, and this included polycystic-appearing ovaries. A diagnosis could be made if two of the following were present:

- Hyperandrogenism (excess of hormones such as testosterone)
- Oligo-anovulation (irregular ovulation)
- Polycystic-appearing ovaries

This dramatically increased the number of people diagnosed with PCOS. Based on the Rotterdam Criteria, PCOS could be diagnosed based on just irregular ovulation and polycystic ovaries, and not excess androgens, which many argue is what defines PCOS.

However, in 2006, the Androgen Excess Society (AES) argued that hyperandrogenism should be essential in diagnosing PCOS. The AES guidelines required hirsutism and/or biochemical hyperandrogenism, and either irregular ovulation or polycystic-appearing ovaries to be present. This criteria excluded those who only had symptoms of irregular ovulation and polycystic ovaries.

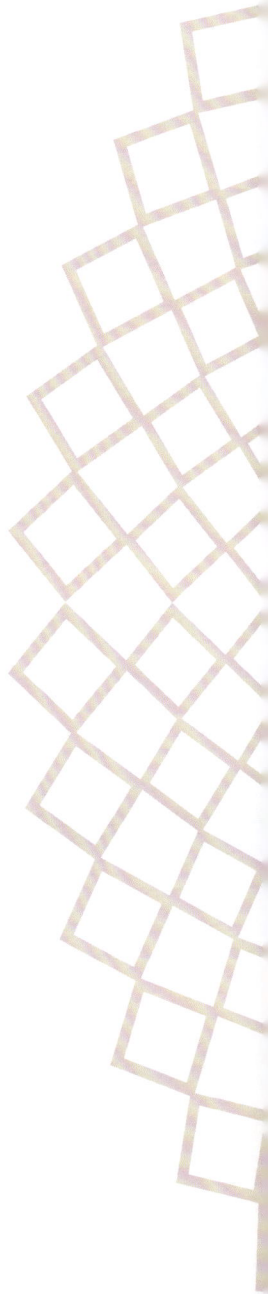

Without making matters more confusing, based on the above diagnostic criteria, you can have polycystic ovaries (PCO) and not polycystic ovary syndrome (PCOS), and you can have PCOS, but not have PCO. This means that to obtain a PCOS diagnosis, globally, an ultrasound alone to determine PCO not enough – it must be accompanied by a blood test and clinical evaluation of symptoms.

Anti-Müllerian hormone (AMH) may also be taken into consideration when diagnosing PCOS. AMH is secreted by ovarian follicles. Due to higher amounts of ovarian follicles, those with PCOS may present with higher levels of AMH.

The more we learn about PCOS, the more apparent it is that each case looks different. You may have a friend with PCOS whose symptoms are different to yours and may respond differently to medications or lifestyle changes. This may be due to different underlying drivers, which has led to differing classifications for those with the condition, depending on their individual characteristics.

If it isn't PCOS, what is it?

There are other disorders that may present similar symptoms to PCOS. This may include Hypothalamic Amenorrhea (HA), in which ovulation (and therefore menstruation) is absent, often due to chronic stress, including undereating and/or over-exercising. In both PCOS and HA, we may see absent periods and even signs of androgen excess. However, in PCOS, blood tests may present a higher ratio of LH:FSH, and low SHBG compared to high SHBG in HA. Healthcare providers may perform something called a progesterone challenge to differentiate between the two. This is when a synthetic progestin is given. If it stimulates a withdrawal bleed, it is indicative of PCOS. If not, HA may be the reason for the missing periods.

Other conditions include hypothyroidism or hyperthyroidism, high prolactin levels, and non-classical congenital adrenal hyperplasia. Those with PCOS can also have an underactive thyroid, and it can be common to see both.

PCOS Complications

If unmanaged, PCOS is associated with an increased risk of developing certain health conditions. These include type 2 diabetes and cardiovascular disease, the umbrella term for anything that impacts the heart or blood vessels, including high blood pressure and high cholesterol.

PCOS is the leading cause of infertility globally (although this is treatable) and may increase complications during pregnancy, including gestational diabetes and pre-eclampsia.

If regular menstruation is not occurring, there may also be an increased risk of endometrial cancer. Those with PCOS are also more likely to experience mental health issues, such as eating disorders, depression and anxiety. This can all feel rather overwhelming and scary, but hope is not lost. While there is no cure for PCOS, understanding your condition can help you take control of the symptoms.

Can Diet Help to Manage PCOS Symptoms?

It can be frustrating to learn that PCOS cannot be cured. However, it can absolutely be managed, and symptoms reduced. In fact, diet is well-recognized as an effective tool for managing PCOS, helping to regulate insulin production and blood glucose levels, therefore reducing symptoms and complications.

If you have PCOS, you may have been told that losing weight will help to improve symptoms and decrease the risk of developing associated conditions. However, while this is true, it can be frustrating to hear, especially as weight gain or difficulty losing weight is a symptom of PCOS. This can be down to insulin resistance, so improving insulin resistance and being mindful of overall energy expenditure and calorie intake will likely have more impact than primarily focusing on the latter.

A PCOS-Friendly Diet

So, what does a PCOS-friendly diet look like? And is it the same for every person with PCOS?

Research strongly suggests that it can help to keep carbohydrate consumption low, with some studies even showing promising results with the keto diet (very low carbohydrate, high fat).

This is because insulin resistance sits at the root of most cases of PCOS, and excess intake of simple carbohydrates and refined sugars worsens insulin resistance. As a result, we remain in that loop of high insulin, impaired glucose tolerance, and an overproduction of androgens. Breaking that cycle means reducing insulin levels, which can be achieved through mindful carbohydrate consumption and reducing sugar intake.

Addressing the insulin component to your PCOS is key, even if you are a healthy weight. You can have insulin resistance and not experience weight gain or difficulty maintaining a healthy weight.

CARBOHYDRATES

Everybody's carbohydrate tolerance is different, and this very much depends on your individual needs, including activity levels. While very low-carb diets, such as keto and even practices like intermittent fasting, do show an improvement in symptoms, this doesn't mean that it is suitable for everyone.

What's more, we need to factor in the nutrients that may be lost from diets like the keto diet, such as fibre, which is found in many complex carbohydrates, making it potentially challenging to be on a very low-carb diet and get adequate fibre.

The benefits of fibre go far beyond just healthy digestive function. It supports metabolic health, cardiovascular health and has even been shown to benefit weight loss, if that is your goal.

Based on those benefits, we can say that fibre is pretty important when it comes to PCOS!

If you are newly diagnosed, first think about the quality of your carbs, rather than no carbs. Swap to carbohydrates that are in their whole, unprocessed form, such as wholegrains, legumes, fruits, vegetables and potatoes. These have their fibre still intact compared to refined carbohydrates, such as white bread and pastries. The more fibre a carbohydrate contains, the slower the digestion of the glucose that naturally occurs in the food, meaning less insulin is released.

You may want to consider slowly reducing overall carbohydrate intake while still being mindful of opting for complex, fibrous carbs when they do appear on your plate. Choose a wholemeal bun for a homemade burger instead of potatoes on the side, or reduce your portion of rice and add in shredded non-starchy vegetables, such as cauliflower or broccoli, for extra bulk.

PROTEIN

Protein is widely known for its muscle-maintaining benefits, which is important to consider for PCOS, as muscle mass increases insulin sensitivity. Protein also helps to keep you feeling satiated.

Current recommended daily protein requirements for women are on the lower end and don't necessarily factor in individual activity levels or the fact that we lose muscle mass as we age. A good way to approach protein, if you are new to thinking about your intake, is to first and foremost ensure that there is a source present in every meal, and then slowly increase from there depending on your personal needs and how satiated you feel after each meal. If you are hungry an hour later or don't feel like your resistance training is giving you the desired effects, eat more protein!

FATS

Fat is the backbone of our hormones, with cholesterol being the precursor. This means that without adequate fat, we run the risk of hormone imbalances and suboptimal hormone levels. A number of our vitamins, specifically A, D, E and K, require fat for absorption. Including healthy fats on your plate also helps to promote satiety, keeping you feeling fuller for longer.

Not all fats are created equal, and this can be where things get confusing. As a rule of thumb, aim for whole, unprocessed fat sources. Focus primarily on monounsaturated fats (such as avocado), polyunsaturated fats (nuts and seeds) and small amounts of saturated fats (butter). Trans fats are found in ultra-processed foods and should be kept to a minimum. This also goes for foods fried in seed oils that have been reheated over and over, as during the heating process, molecules in the oils can become unstable and problematic in the body.

There are also omega-3, essential fatty acids, which include EPA, DHA and ALA. We convert a very small amount of ALA (found in nuts and seeds) into EPA and DHA. Fish, which is rich in DHA and EPA, is by far the superior form of this type of omega-3. Omega-3 supports a healthy cardiovascular system, key for PCOS, and some research shows it may lower androgens and insulin levels.

MICRONUTRIENTS

Fat, protein and carbohydrates make up your macronutrients, while vitamins, minerals and plant compounds, such as polyphenols, are micronutrients. Whole, unprocessed foods will often have a higher micronutrient profile, and the more variety of plants and animal-based proteins you include in your diet, the more diverse your intake of micronutrients will be.

Different vitamins and minerals will help different processes in the body. For example, iron, found in animal protein and dark leafy greens, is crucial for optimal energy levels as it transports oxygen around the body. Zinc, found in shellfish and pumpkin seeds, supports the immune system, and can help to regulate androgens.

Certain foods also contain compounds that have antioxidant properties. This can help to combat oxidative stress in the body, which is known to increase inflammation and complications related to PCOS.

The Mediterranean diet is one of the most widely studied diets and for good reason. For PCOS, it seems like the obvious choice due to the prevalence of antioxidant-rich plants, healthy fats and whole, unprocessed carbohydrates. For example, one study found that a low-carb Mediterranean diet helped to restore menstrual cycles and hormone levels in overweight PCOS patients, and was significantly more effective than a low-fat diet.

The inclusion of polyphenols (plant compounds) and adequate fibre in our diet also helps to maintain and feed the different colonies of bacteria that live in our gut. A healthy gut microbiome is linked to healthy immune function, mental wellbeing and metabolic health, all of which are important for managing PCOS. Those with PCOS may have an imbalance of bacteria in the gut microbiome, driving chronic inflammation.

The Best Diet for You

Labels aside, when considering the way you eat to manage your PCOS, the perfect diet is the one that not only improves your individual symptoms, but one that you can maintain for the rest of your life. It shouldn't feel restrictive or isolating. As PCOS is a condition that has to be managed long-term, you therefore need to think about a long-term approach to your nutrition.

PCOS Diet Golden Rules

PCOS DIET STAPLES

- Oily fish, such as salmon, sardines and mackerel
- Lean proteins, such as chicken and turkey
- Beef and lamb
- Eggs
- Fermented dairy, including yogurt and kefir
- Healthy fats, including olive oil and avocado
- Nuts and seeds
- Dark leafy green vegetables, such as spinach, chard and rocket
- Colourful, non-starchy vegetables, such as peppers, courgettes and broccoli
- Berries and cherries
- Apples and pears
- Fermented vegetables, such as sauerkraut and kimchi
- Wholegrains, including quinoa, brown rice and buckwheat
- Legumes, such as beans and lentils
- Anti-inflammatory spices, such as turmeric, ginger and cinnamon
- Cacao and dark chocolate
- Green tea, spearmint tea and nettle tea

FOODS TO AVOID / KEEP TO A MINIMUM

- Refined carbohydrates, including white bread, cakes, pastries and white-flour pasta
- Sugary desserts, cereals and processed snacks
- Alcohol
- Fried foods and snacks, such as crisps
- Margarine
- Processed and barbecued meats
- Sugary drinks, such as sodas and fruit juice
- Dried fruits

Beyond Food:
PCOS Lifestyle Changes

While good nutrition is a foundational pillar for effectively managing PCOS symptoms, we can't ignore the positive impact that the right lifestyle changes can also have.

EXERCISE

The impact that exercise can have on both our mental and cardiovascular health is well known, but exercise can be another tool for your PCOS toolkit to aid insulin sensitivity. Resistance training and building muscle mass in particular can help to reduce insulin resistance that may be driving hyperandrogenism (excess facial and body hair), and can help to increase metabolic rate.

SLEEP

Optimizing sleep quality is another important lifestyle consideration. Poor sleep quality can impact our stress hormones, which drive blood sugar imbalances and inflammation. You are also more likely to snack and experience an increase in cravings when you are sleep-deprived, so putting a good night's sleep at the top of your priority list can help with PCOS symptoms and reduce risk factors.

STRESS

Stress may look different for everyone. From work stress and finances to nutrient deficiencies and illness, stress can exacerbate the hormonal imbalances occurring in PCOS, making it harder to manage symptoms. Stress, unfortunately, is part of modern-day life, and is hard to avoid completely.

What matters, however, is your perception of that stress. Reducing the stress that you can control, and effectively managing the stressors that you can't, is the best way to approach it and will help to effectively manage PCOS symptoms and reduce complications.

SUPPLEMENTS

There are a number of evidence-based supplements that can be another valuable addition to your PCOS toolkit. They do not replace the need for a well-rounded, balanced diet, but they may help to fill in any gaps. Supplements should do what the name suggests: supplement an already solid PCOS diet and lifestyle protocol.

It is important to always consult your healthcare provider before starting a new supplement routine, as certain nutrients or herbs may interact with medications.

The most widely studied supplements for PCOS include:

- Zinc
- Vitamin D
- Inositol (a combination of myo-inositol and d-chiro inositol)
- Turmeric or curcumin
- Omega-3 or fish oil
- N-acetyl cysteine (NAC)
- CoQ10
- Vitamin E
- Magnesium

MEDICATIONS

The health and wellness industry can feel quite polarizing at times, and we're flooded with extreme opinions from every direction. There is no downside to optimizing your diet to support your PCOS, and if you feel as though you need extra support, certain medications – always discussed in consultation with your doctor – may give you that helping hand you need.

Common medications for PCOS include metformin, which lowers blood sugar, and spironolactone, which blocks androgen receptors. Glucagon-like peptide-1 receptor agonists may also be recommended as part of a PCOS treatment plan to aid with weight loss and insulin resistance.

The oral contraceptive pill may be recommended by your doctor if periods are missing, which artificially forces the shedding of your uterus lining when you take a week's break, reducing your risks of certain cancers. The type of progestin in oral contraceptives has anti-androgen action, too. If you are trying to conceive, you may be recommended drugs to support your ovulation by your doctor or fertility specialist.

A Final Thought

While this recipe book should leave you feeling excited and inspired about maintaining a PCOS-friendly lifestyle, it is not meant to replace advice from your doctor. When making any nutrition changes, seek professional advice from your doctor.

Breakfast & Brunch

Quinoa Porridge
with Raspberries

Your gut microbiome loves variety and a healthy, diverse gut microbiome is not only associated with good cardiometabolic health, it also plays a role in regulating your mood and energy levels. All of these are key considerations when it comes to eating for PCOS and reducing risk factors. Mixing up your wholegrains, such as swapping oats for quinoa, is a great way to increase plant diversity and nourish your gut microbiome.

SERVES **2**

600 ml (1 pint) milk

100 g (3½ oz) quinoa

½ teaspoon ground cinnamon

125 g (4 oz) fresh raspberries

2 tablespoons mixed seeds (pumpkin, hemp, sunflower, sesame, linseed)

1 tablespoon clear honey

1 Bring the milk to the boil in a small saucepan. Add the quinoa and return the mixture to the boil, then reduce the heat to low, cover and simmer for about 15 minutes until three-quarters of the milk has been absorbed.

2 Stir the cinnamon into the pan, re-cover and cook for 8–10 minutes, or until almost all the milk has been absorbed and the quinoa is tender.

3 Spoon the porridge into 2 bowls, then top with the raspberries, sprinkle over the seeds and drizzle with the honey. Serve immediately.

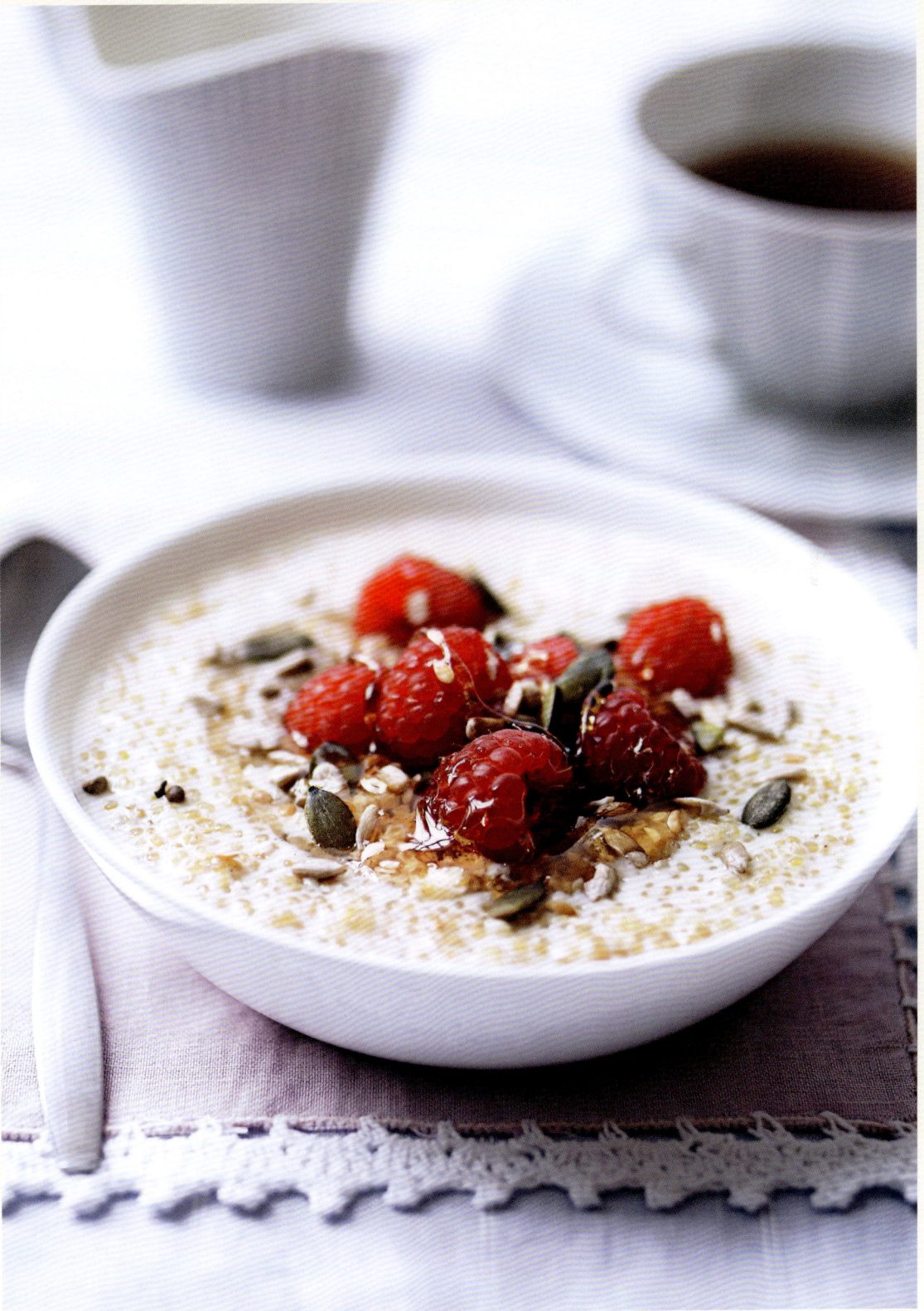

Granola
with Chocolate Chips

Making your own granola is a great way to avoid added sugar in your diet, plus you can add as many nutrient-dense, high-fibre extras (such as nuts and seeds) as you wish. These fibrous extras help to maintain a healthy and diverse gut microbiome and keep your blood sugar levels stable.

SERVES 1

3 tablespoons jumbo porridge oats

1 tablespoon hazelnuts

1 tablespoon pistachio nuts

1 tablespoon mixed seeds (pumpkin, hemp, sunflower, sesame, linseed)

2 teaspoons light olive oil

2 teaspoons clear honey

TO SERVE

150 ml (¼ pint) natural yogurt

2 tablespoons fresh pomegranate seeds

2 teaspoons plain dark chocolate chips

1 Heat a large nonstick frying pan. Toss the oats, hazelnuts, pistachio nuts and mixed seeds in the pan for a couple of minutes until lightly toasted.

2 Add the olive oil and honey to the mixture and stir everything together.

3 Tip into a bowl and top with the yogurt, pomegranate seeds and chocolate chips for a delicious breakfast.

tip | Serve with Greek yogurt for a protein boost.

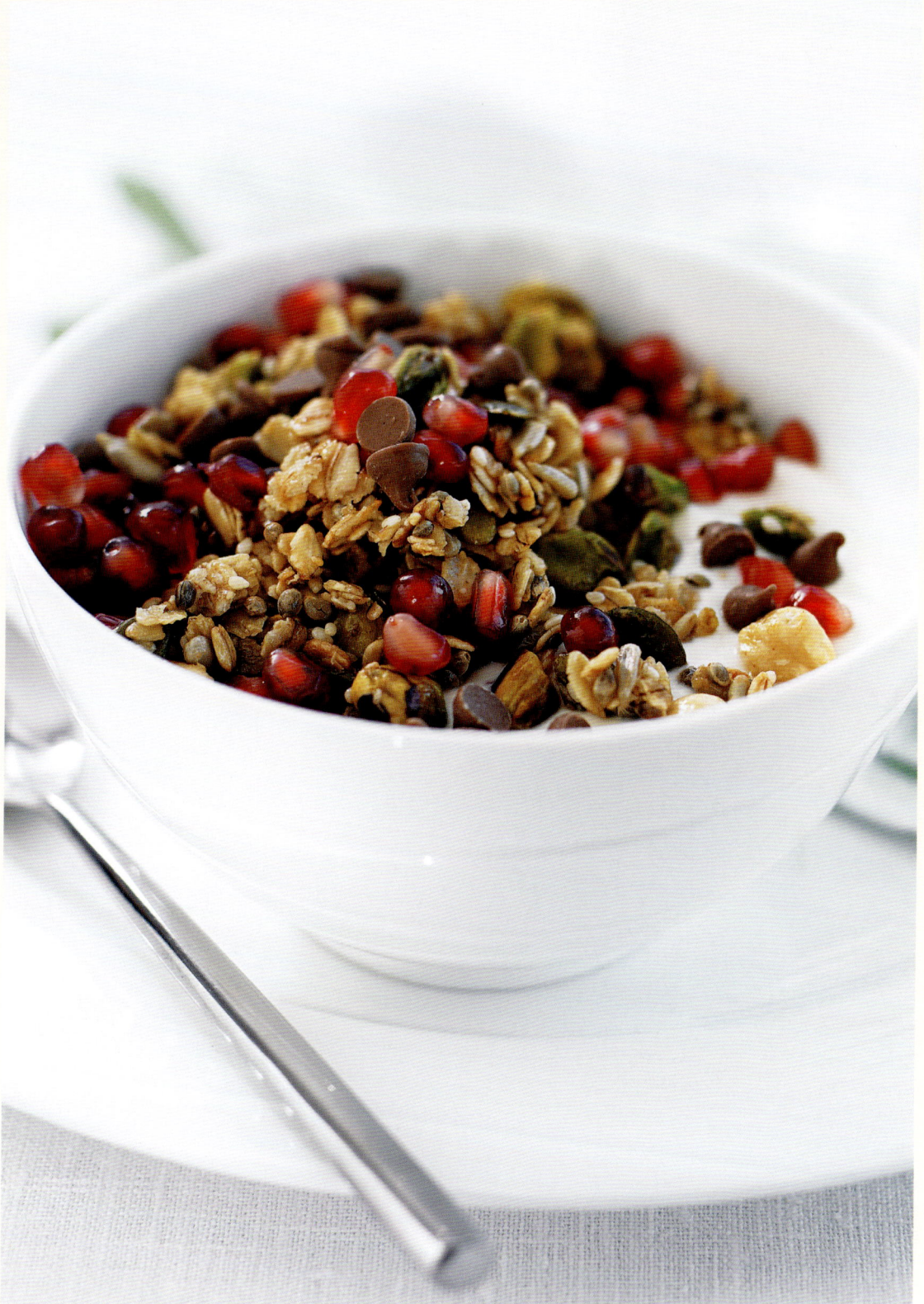

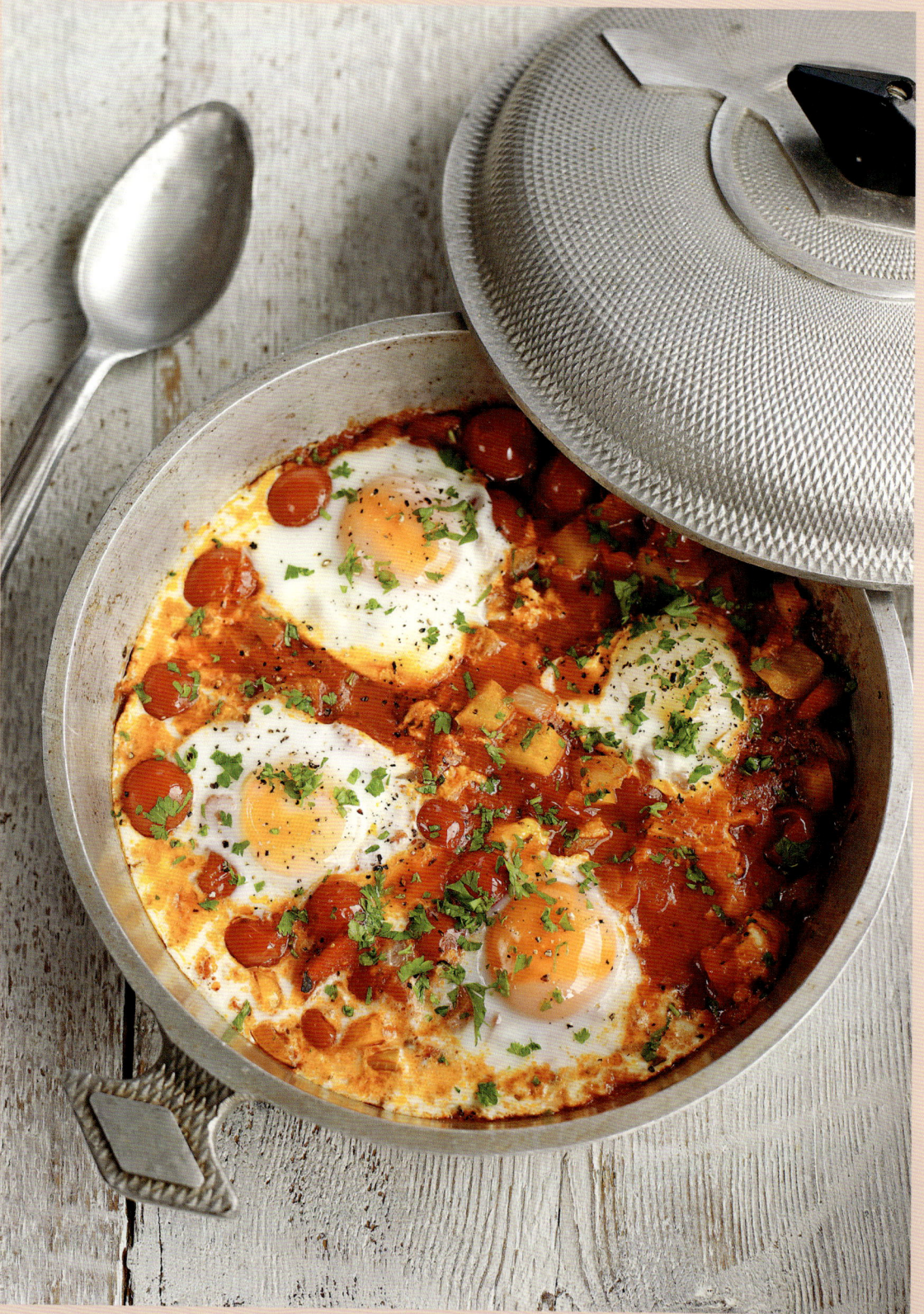

Ranch-style Eggs

This makes the perfect slow Sunday brunch. Baking eggs in tomato sauce and spices means not only do you elevate the flavour but you boost the nutrition, too. This recipe is low in carbs, but high in protein and fibre, guaranteed to keep blood sugar levels stable and prevent energy crashes later on in the day.

SERVES **2**

2 tablespoons olive oil

1 onion, finely sliced

1 red chilli, deseeded and
    finely chopped

1 garlic clove, crushed

1 teaspoon ground cumin

1 teaspoon dried oregano

400 g (13 oz) canned cherry tomatoes

200 g (7 oz) roasted red and yellow
    peppers in oil (from a jar), drained
    and roughly chopped

4 eggs

salt and pepper

4 tablespoons finely chopped coriander,
    to garnish

1   Heat the oil in a large frying pan and add the onion, chilli, garlic, cumin and oregano. Fry gently for about 5 minutes or until soft.

2   Add the tomatoes and peppers and cook for a further 5 minutes. If the sauce looks dry, add a splash of water.

3   Season well and make 4 hollows in the mixture. Break an egg into each hollow, then cover the pan. Cook for 5 minutes or until the eggs are just set.

4   Serve immediately, garnished with the chopped coriander.

Chickpea & Spinach Omelette

If chickpeas aren't already a staple in your pantry, that needs to change! Chickpeas make a versatile addition to most types of dishes, providing a slow release of energy due to the ratio of fibre to carbohydrates, and also providing plant-based protein. They are a fabulous source of vitamin B6, which helps the body produce serotonin, a neurotransmitter that regulates our mood.

SERVES 4

2 tablespoons olive oil

1 large onion, sliced

1 red pepper, sliced

½ teaspoon hot smoked or sweet paprika

400 g (13 oz) can chickpeas, drained and rinsed

100 g (3½ oz) spinach leaves, rinsed and roughly sliced

5 eggs, lightly beaten

75 g (3 oz) pitted green olives, roughly chopped

150 g (5 oz) Cheddar cheese, grated

salt and pepper

1 Heat the olive oil in a large nonstick frying pan. Add the onion and pepper and cook gently for 7–8 minutes, until soft and golden.

2 Stir in the paprika and chickpeas and cook for 1 minute, stirring frequently. Add the spinach leaves and cook until just wilted.

3 Pour the beaten eggs into the pan and stir to combine. Cook gently, without stirring, for 4–5 minutes until almost set.

4 Sprinkle with the olives and grated Cheddar, then slide under a preheated hot grill, keeping the handle away from the heat. Grill for 4–5 minutes until golden and set. Slice into wedges and serve immediately.

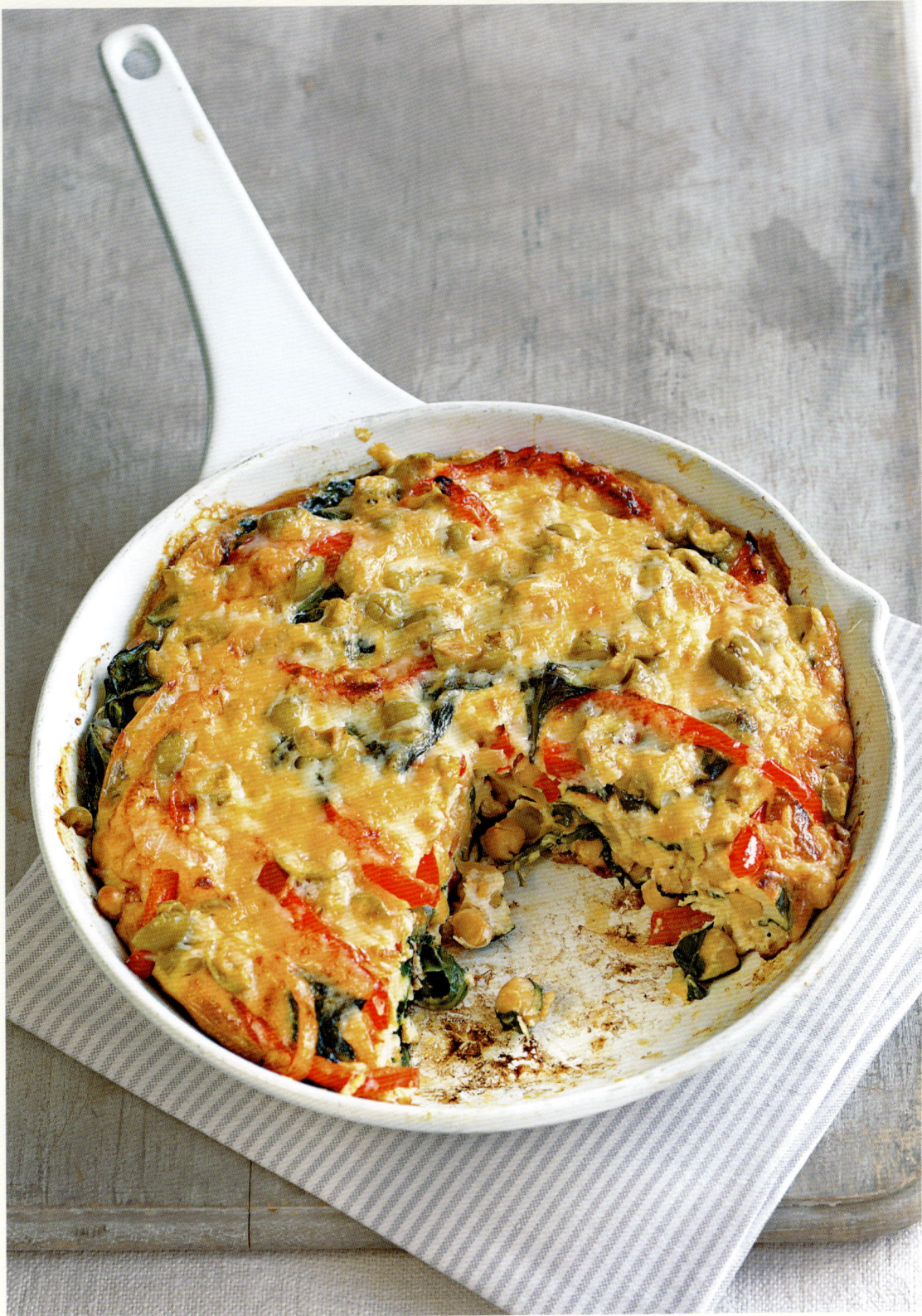

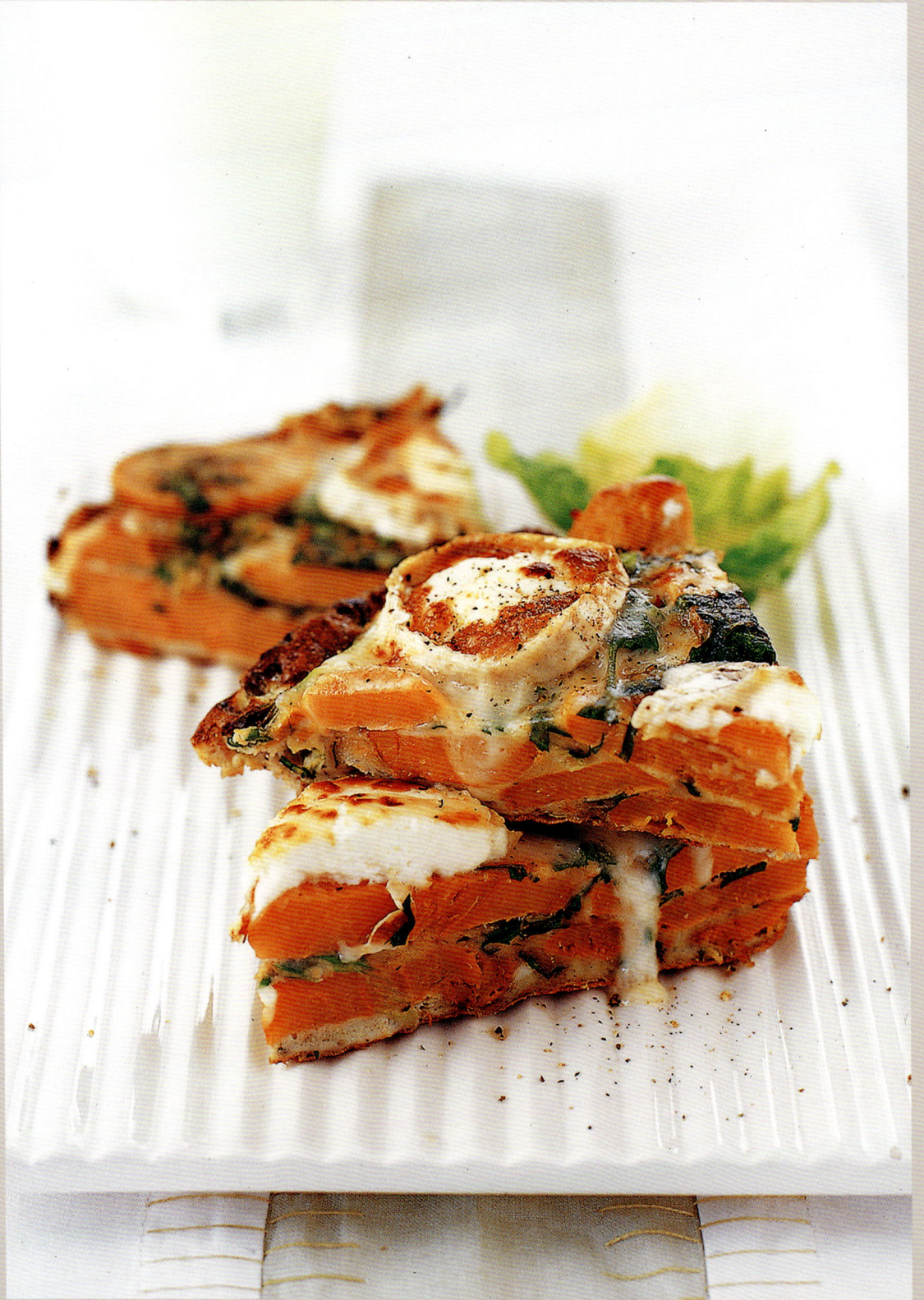

Sweet Potato & Cheese Frittata

Short on time in the morning? A frittata is the perfect solution. You can do all the prep and cooking ahead of time, and then take it on the go. If you eat this frittata cold, or even if you reheat it, by cooling it beforehand you will have increased the amount of resistant starch the sweet potato contains. Resistant starch not only feeds the good bugs in your gut, but has little impact on blood sugar levels, making it a great hack for PCOS.

SERVES **4**

500 g (1 lb) sweet potatoes, sliced
1 teaspoon olive oil
5 spring onions, sliced
2 tablespoons chopped fresh coriander
4 large eggs, beaten
100 g (3½ oz) round goats' cheese with
    rind, cut into 4 slices
pepper

1 Put the sweet potato slices in a saucepan of boiling water and cook for 7–8 minutes, or until just tender, then drain.

2 Heat the oil in a medium nonstick frying pan, add the spring onions and sweet potato slices and fry for 2 minutes.

3 Stir the coriander into the beaten eggs, season with plenty of pepper and pour into the pan. Arrange the slices of goats' cheese on top and continue to cook for 3–4 minutes until almost set.

4 Put the pan under a preheated hot grill and cook for 2–3 minutes until golden and bubbling. Serve immediately.

tip | Add a handful of leafy greens of your choosing on the side to really boost the nutrition profile! Rocket works great here.

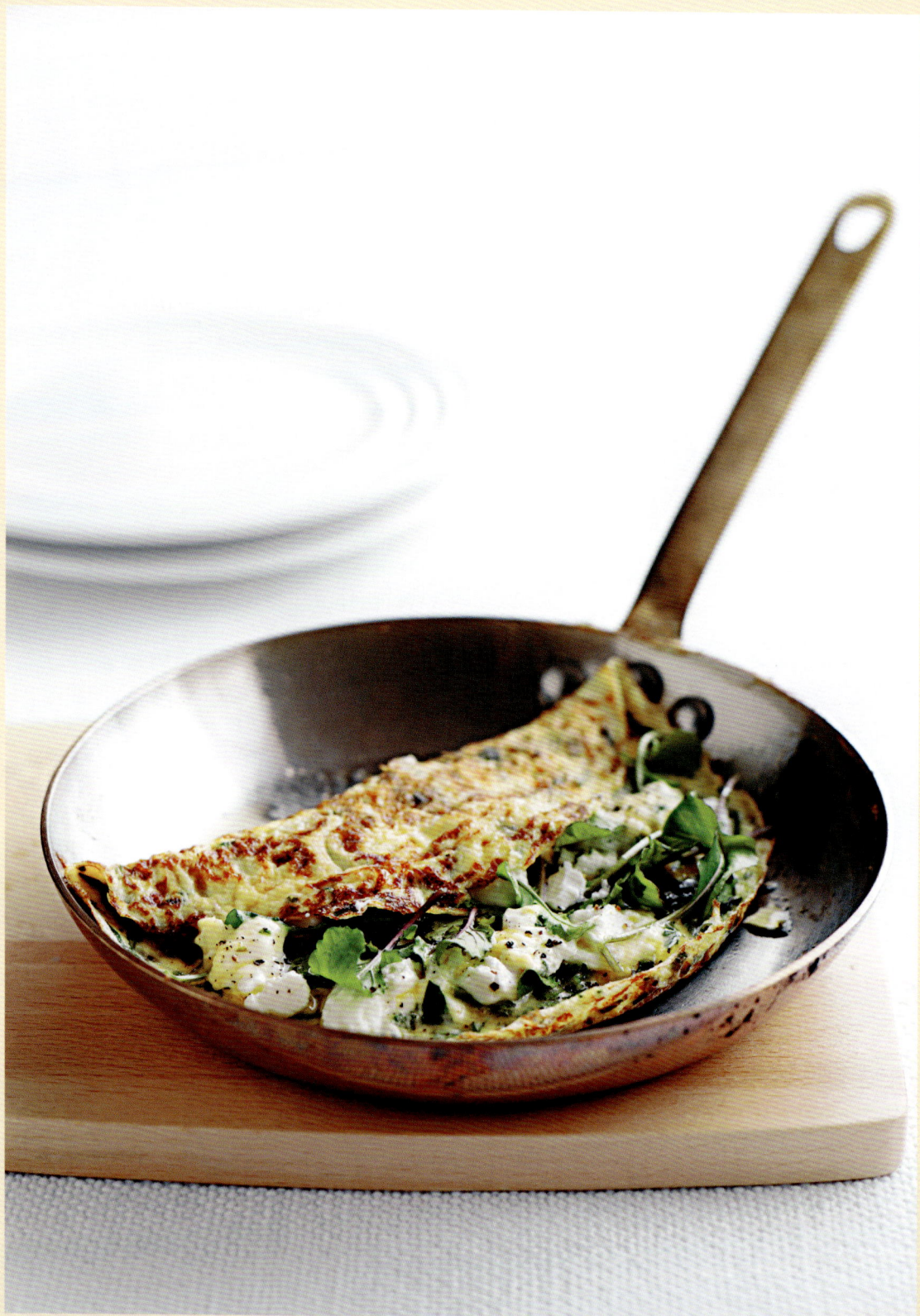

Rocket & Goats' Cheese Omelette

This herby, green omelette will set you up perfectly for the day ahead. It doesn't take long to make, but the high protein content will keep you satiated and prevent dips later on, helping you take on whatever the day throws at you.

SERVES **4**

12 eggs

4 tablespoons milk

4 tablespoons chopped mixed herbs,
    such as chervil, chives, marjoram,
    parsley and tarragon

2 tablespoons olive oil

125 g (4 oz) soft goats' cheese, diced

small handful of baby rocket leaves

salt and pepper

1   Beat the eggs, milk and herbs together in a large bowl along with some salt and pepper.

2   Heat the olive oil in an omelette pan, then swirl in a quarter of the egg mixture. Cook over a medium heat, forking over the omelette so that it cooks evenly.

3   As soon as the omelette is set on the underside, but still a little runny in the centre, scatter a quarter of the cheese and a quarter of the rocket leaves over one half of the omelette. Carefully slide the omelette on to a warmed serving plate, folding it in half as you go. For the best results, serve immediately.

4   Repeat to make 3 more omelettes and serve each individually. Alternatively, keep warm in a moderate oven and serve together.

Butternut Squash & Ricotta Frittata

Butternut squash really deserves a place on your PCOS grocery list! Its high fibre content helps with glycemic control and insulin sensitivity, and its texture in a frittata almost mimics that of potato, but with an added natural sweetness that pairs perfectly with ricotta.

SERVES **6**

1 tablespoon olive oil

1 red onion, thinly sliced

450 g (14½ oz) peeled and deseeded
    butternut squash, diced

8 eggs

2 tablespoons chopped sage

1 tablespoon chopped thyme

125 g (4 oz) ricotta cheese

salt and pepper

1   Heat the oil in a large, deep frying pan with an ovenproof handle over a medium-low heat. Add the onion and butternut squash, then cover loosely and cook gently, stirring frequently, for 18–20 minutes until softened and golden.

2   Lightly beat together the eggs, herbs and ricotta in a jug, then season well with salt and pepper.

3   Pour the egg mixture over the squash mixture and cook for 2–3 minutes until the egg is almost set, stirring occasionally to prevent the base from burning.

4   Slide the pan under a preheated hot grill, keeping the handle away from the heat, and cook for 3–4 minutes until the egg is set and the frittata is golden.

5   Slice into 6 wedges and serve hot.

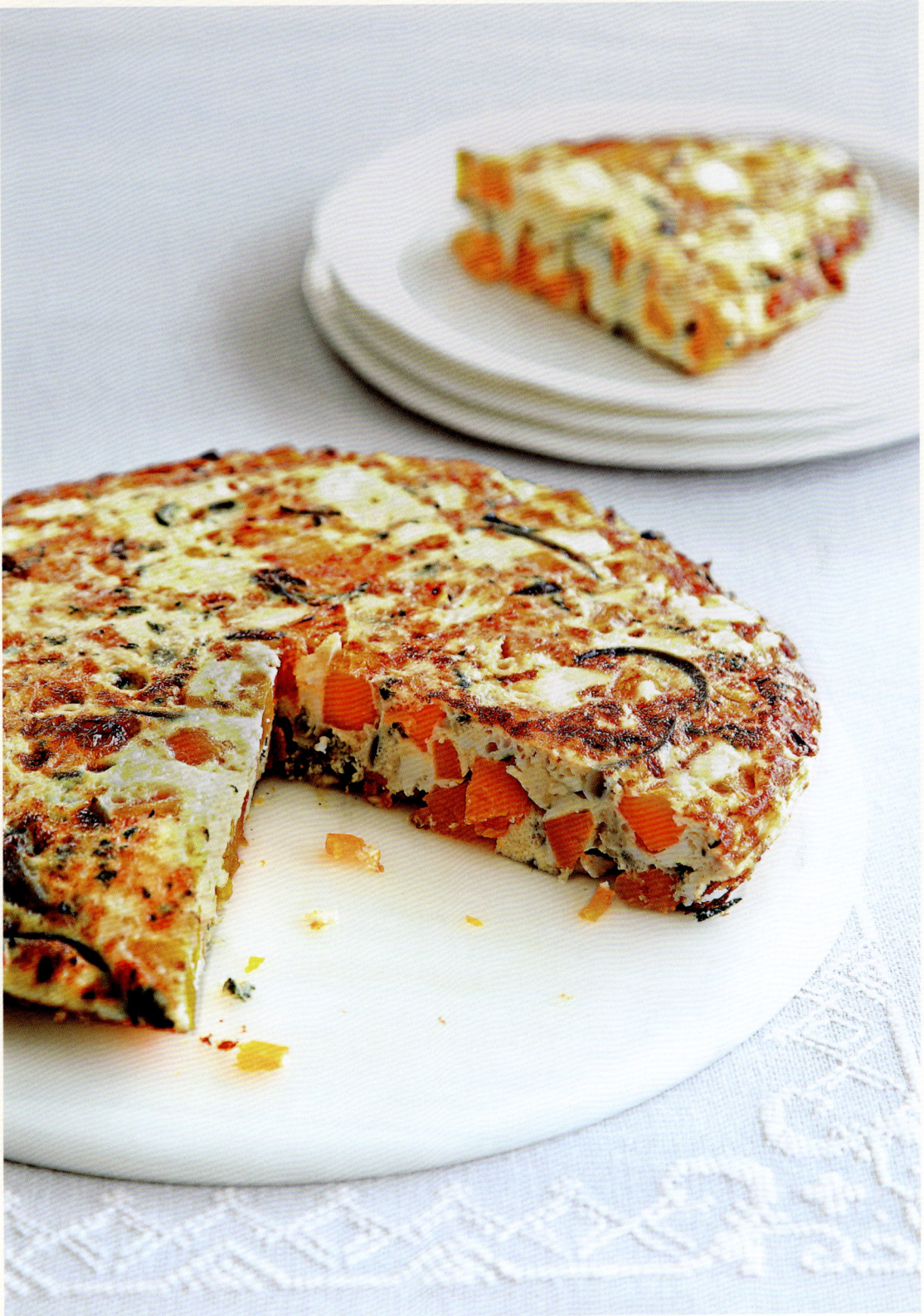

All-in-One Veggie Breakfast

This all-in-one dish is a delicious way to tick off all three of the macronutrients needed to keep you feeling your best throughout the morning. The beauty of this recipe is that you can customize it depending on what you have in your kitchen. Add chicken sausage, turkey bacon or halloumi for extra protein, or any veggies you have in the bottom of your refrigerator.

SERVES **4**

500 g (1 lb) cooked potatoes or sweet
    potatoes, cubed
4 tablespoons olive oil
a few thyme sprigs
250 g (8 oz) button mushrooms,
    trimmed
12 cherry tomatoes
4 eggs
salt and pepper
2 tablespoons chopped parsley,
    to garnish

1   Spread the potato cubes out in a roasting tin. Drizzle over half of the oil, scatter over the thyme sprigs and season with salt and pepper. Bake in a preheated oven, 220°C (425°F), Gas Mark 7, for 10 minutes.

2   Stir the potato cubes well, then add the mushrooms to the tin and bake for another 10 minutes.

3   Now add the tomatoes to the tin and bake for a further 10 minutes.

4   Make four hollows in between the vegetables and carefully break an egg into each hollow. Bake for 3–4 minutes until the eggs are set.

5   Garnish with the parsley and serve straight from the tin.

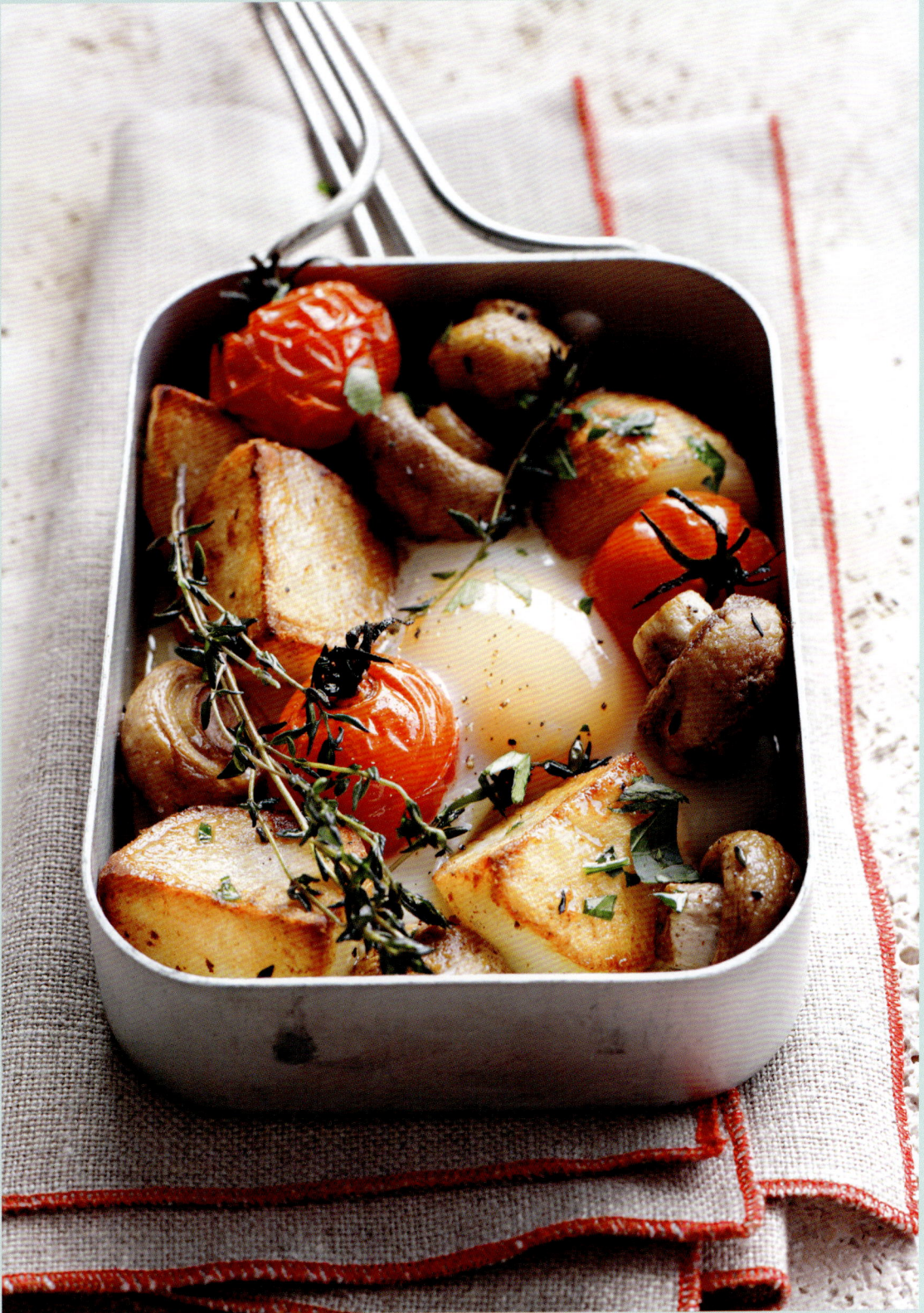

Mushroom Tofu Scramble

When making plant-based meals, it can be easy to forget about the protein. Tofu is a great protein option to include in your veggie or plant-based meals as it is a complete protein source, meaning it contains all nine essential amino acids. By crumbling tofu, you get a lovely, scrambled egg-like texture, that works well combined with mixed vegetables, keeping blood sugar levels stable and you feeling satiated.

SERVES **4**

2 tablespoons olive oil

200 g (7 oz) chestnut mushrooms, trimmed and quartered

250 g (8 oz) firm tofu, drained, patted dry and crumbled

125 g (4 oz) baby plum tomatoes, halved

3 tablespoons chopped flat leaf parsley

salt and pepper

1   Heat the oil in a frying pan, add the mushrooms and cook over a high heat, stirring frequently, for 2 minutes until browned and softened. Add the tofu and cook, stirring, for 1 minute.

2   Add the tomatoes to the pan and cook for 2 minutes until starting to soften. Stir in half of the parsley, then season with salt and pepper.

3   Serve immediately, sprinkled with the remaining parsley.

Breakfast Muesli

By soaking oats overnight, you increase their resistant starch content, which helps to keep blood sugar levels stable. The prebiotic fibre found in oats also helps feed the good bacteria in our guts, while the probiotic-rich yogurt that they are soaked in maintains that bacteria. If you're looking for a gut-healthy, made-ahead-of-time breakfast, this one is for you!

SERVES **2**

125 g (4 oz) jumbo oats
1 tablespoon pumpkin seeds
1 tablespoon sunflower seeds
1 tablespoon sesame seeds
75 g (3 oz) fresh raspberries
50 g (2 oz) fresh blueberries
250 ml (8 fl oz) natural yogurt

TO SERVE

1 tablespoon toasted almonds,
    roughly chopped
2 tablespoons clear honey
milk (optional)

1   Mix together the oats, seeds, berries and yogurt. Chill in the refrigerator overnight.

2   The next day, sprinkle the almonds over and serve the muesli drizzled with the honey, and a little milk, if liked.

tip | Don't have yogurt on hand or want to increase your variety of probiotics? Try kefir in place of the yogurt.

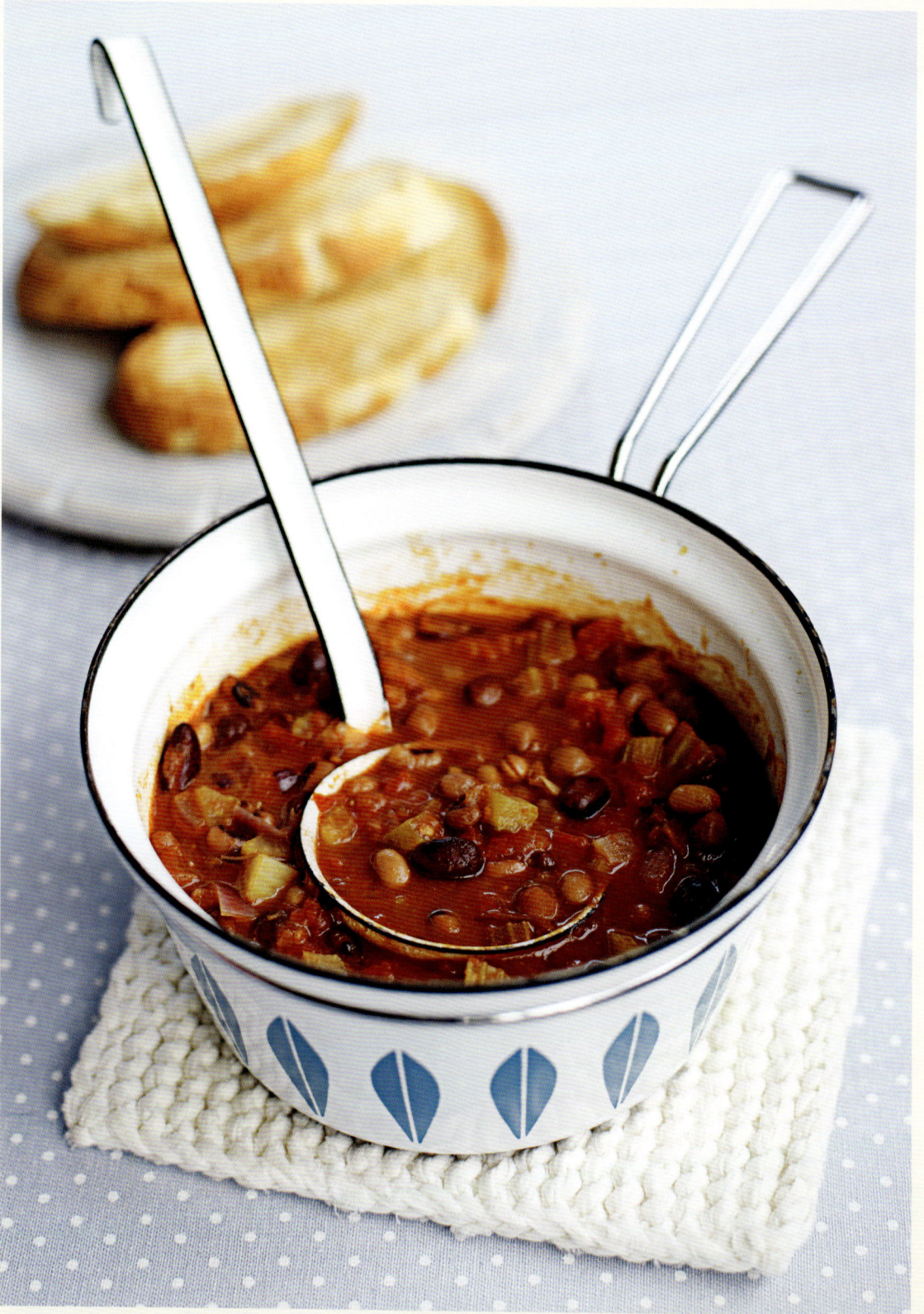

Boston Baked Beans

Beans are a great PCOS staple due to their fibre content. Because of all the fibre, the sugars in the beans are digested more slowly, creating a sustainable release of energy. Instead of grabbing a can of baked beans from the supermarket, spend a little longer in the kitchen and make your own!

SERVES **4**

2 tablespoons olive oil

1 large red onion, finely chopped

4 celery sticks, finely chopped

2 garlic cloves, crushed

400 g (13 oz) can chopped tomatoes

300 ml (½ pint) vegetable stock

2 tablespoons dark soy sauce

4 teaspoons Dijon mustard

2 x 410 g (13½ oz) cans mixed beans, drained and rinsed

4 tablespoons chopped flat leaf parsley

toasted sourdough, to serve

1 Heat the oil in a heavy-based saucepan. Add the onion and cook over a low heat for 5 minutes, or until softened. Add the celery and garlic and continue to cook for 1–2 minutes.

2 Add the tomatoes, stock and soy sauce and bring to the boil, then reduce the heat to a fast simmer and cook for about 15 minutes, or until the sauce begins to thicken.

3 Add the mustard and mixed beans and cook for a further 5 minutes, or until the beans are heated through. Stir in the chopped parsley and serve on toast.

tip | If you need more protein, add a couple of poached eggs or slices of halloumi on top.

Baked Eggs
with Moroccan Spices

Eggs make for the perfect PCOS-friendly breakfast food, as they contain protein and fat. While carbs aren't the enemy, keeping refined carbohydrates (found in many traditional breakfast foods) to a minimum is key for regulating insulin levels and, as a result, reducing many of the symptoms of PCOS.

SERVES **2**

½ tablespoon olive oil
½ onion, chopped
1 garlic clove, sliced
½ teaspoon ras el hanout
pinch of ground cinnamon
½ teaspoon ground coriander
400 g (13 oz) cherry tomatoes
2 tablespoons chopped coriander
2 eggs
salt and pepper

1   Heat the oil in a frying pan over a medium heat. Add the onion and garlic and cook for 6–7 minutes until softened and lightly golden. Stir in the spices and cook, stirring, for 1 minute.

2   Add the tomatoes and season well with salt and pepper. Simmer gently for 8–10 minutes.

3   Scatter over 1 tablespoon of the coriander, then divide the tomato mixture between 2 individual ovenproof dishes. Break an egg into each dish.

4   Bake in a preheated oven, 220°C (425°F), Gas Mark 7, for 8–10 minutes until the egg whites are set but the yolks are still slightly runny. Cook for a further 2–3 minutes if you prefer the eggs to be cooked through.

5   Serve scattered with the remaining coriander.

tip | Serve with some Greek yogurt on the side for more protein!

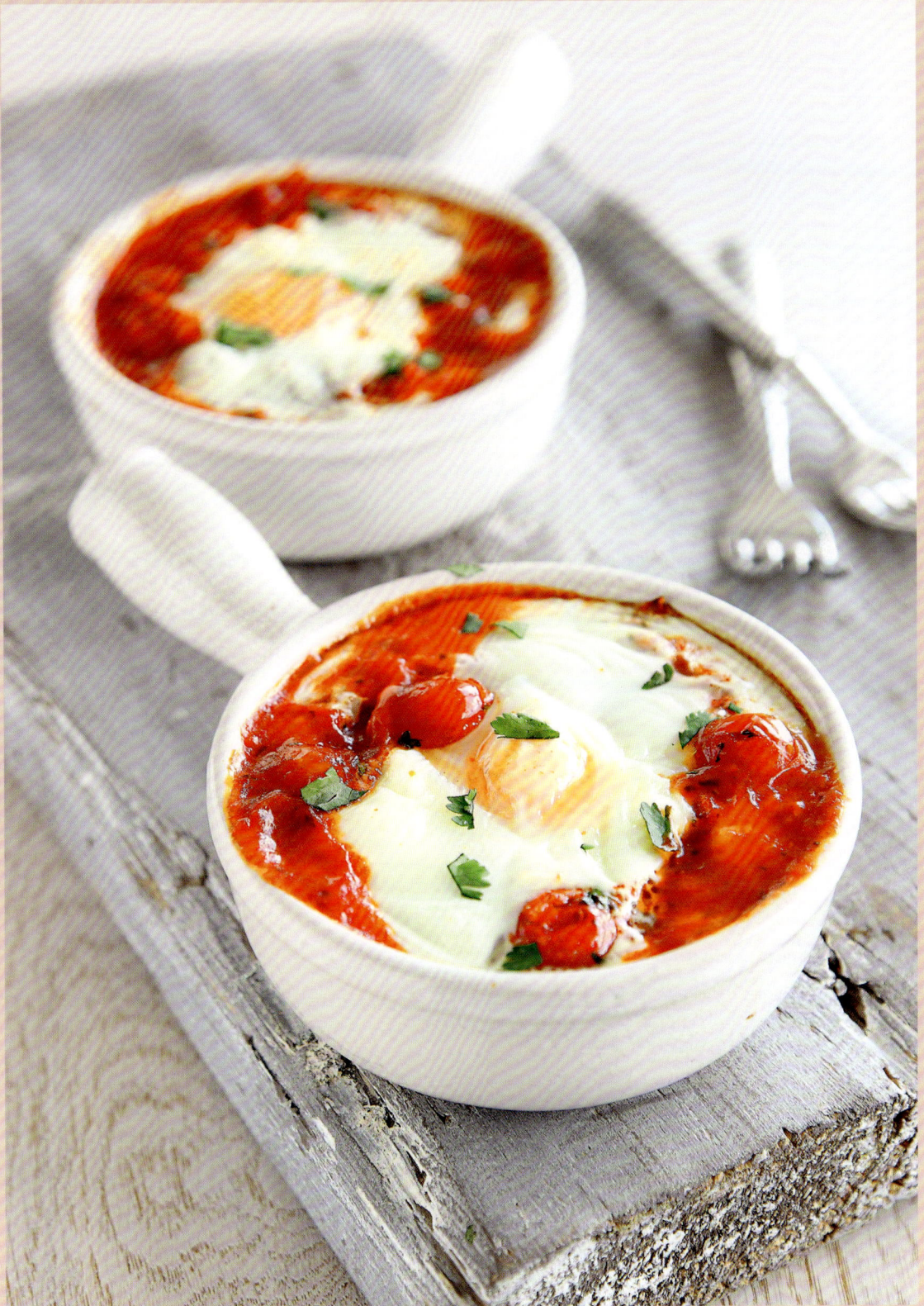

Berry Breakfast

Fast food doesn't have to mean junk food! Yogurt is crammed full of PCOS-friendly micro and macronutrients and makes for a super-speedy breakfast. Add antioxidant-rich, low-sugar, high-fibre berries to the mix and you've further boosted the nutrition profile of the meal.

SERVES **2**

150 ml (½ pint) Greek yogurt
2 teaspoons clear honey
175 g (6 oz) raspberries
15 g (½ oz) porridge oats

1   Put the yogurt in a bowl and fold in the honey.

2   Divide one-third of the raspberries between 2 serving glasses. Cover with half of the yogurt mixture. Scatter over some of the oats and more raspberries, dividing them evenly among the glasses.

3   Repeat the layers, finishing with oats and a few raspberries. Chill in the refrigerator for 30 minutes before serving.

tip | Want to further boost your fibre intake? Scatter flax, hemp or pumpkin seeds over the yogurt alongside the oats.

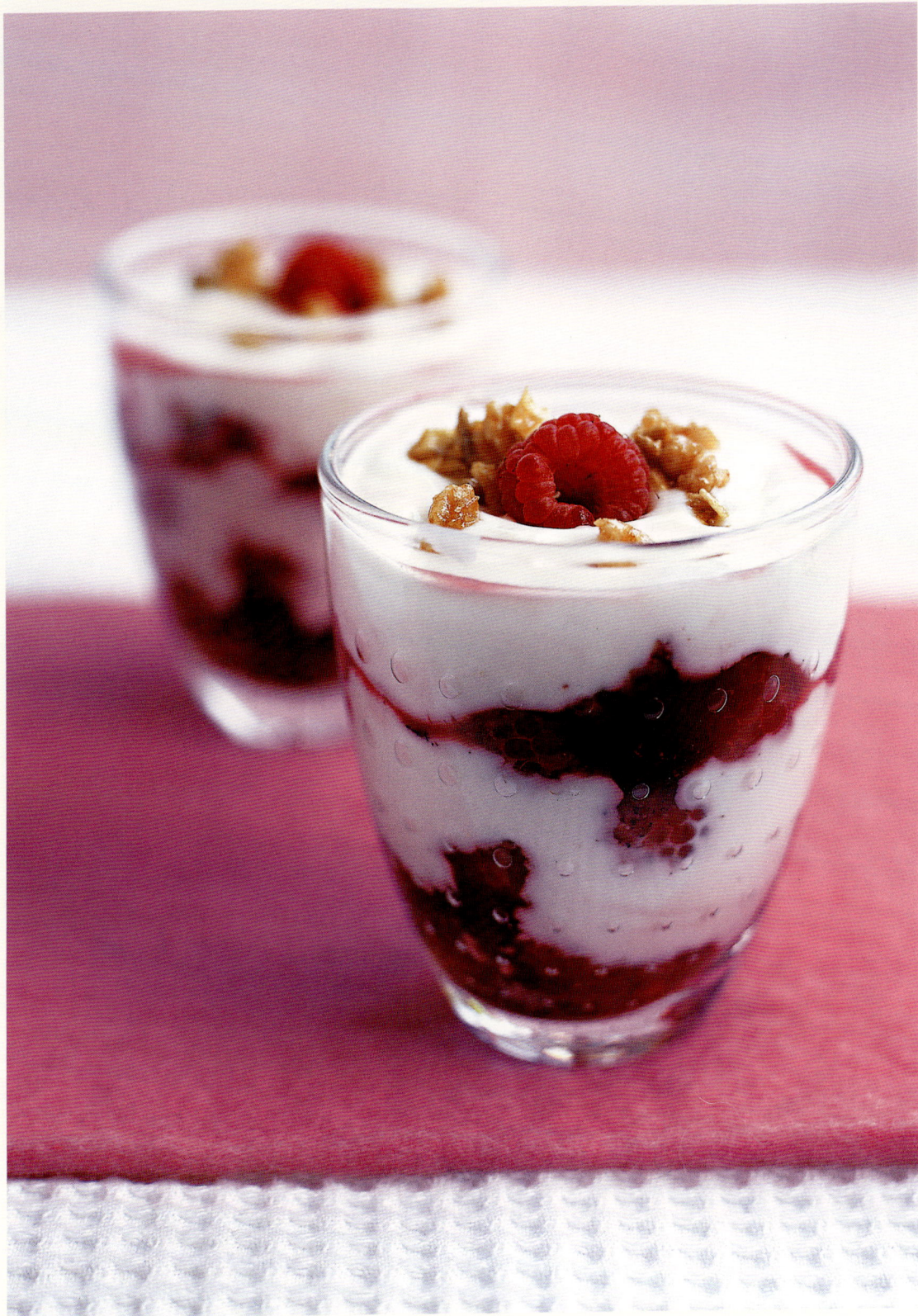

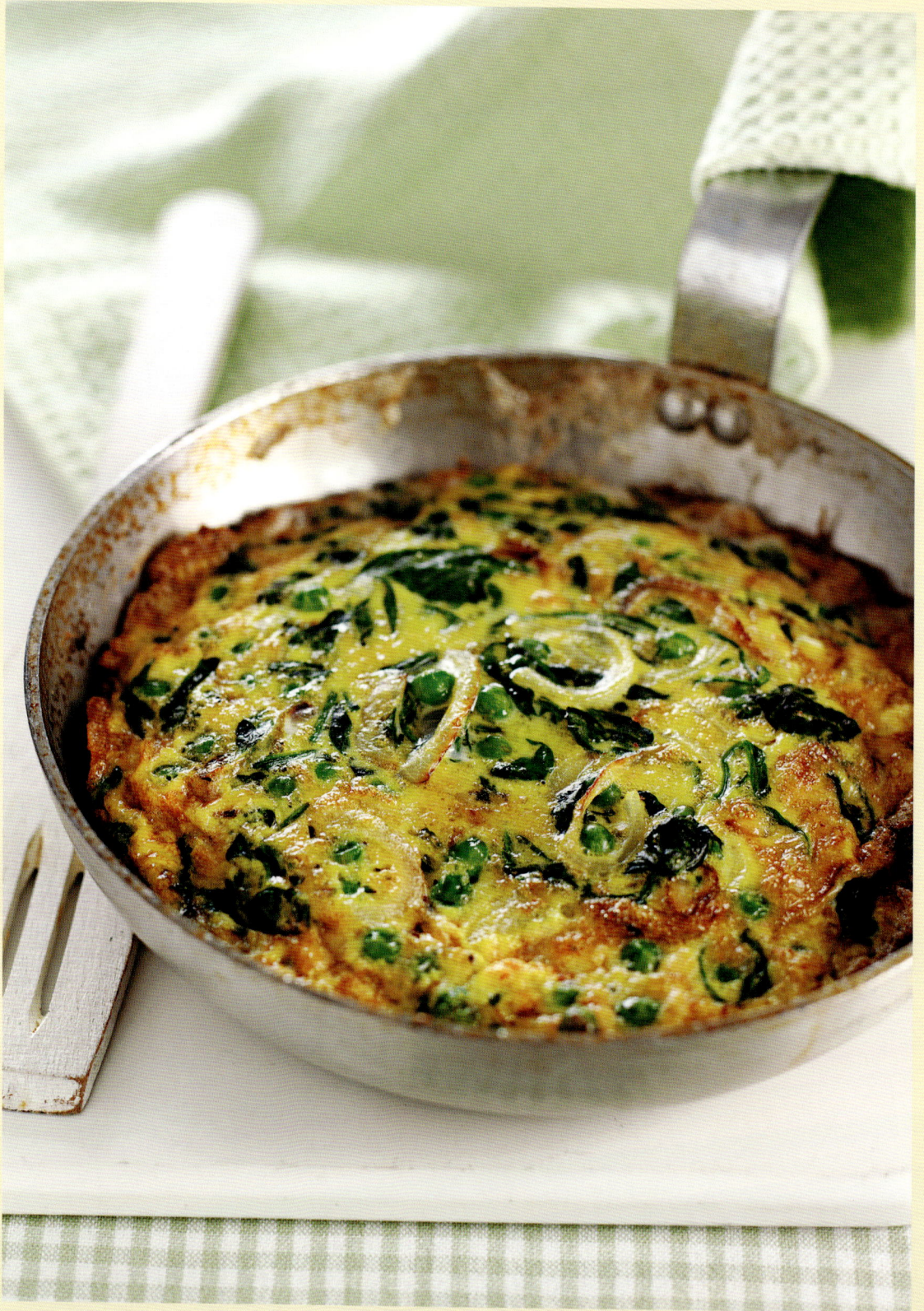

Spinach & Pea Frittata

Dark leafy green vegetables, such as spinach, chard and rocket, are incredibly nutrient-dense and deserve their place on every plate. If you're not a huge fan, hiding them in egg-based dishes or even in smoothies is a great way to reap the benefits.

SERVES **2**

1 tablespoon olive oil
1 onion, thinly sliced
150 g (5 oz) baby spinach
125 g (4 oz) shelled fresh or frozen peas
6 eggs
salt and pepper

1   Heat the oil in a heavy-based, ovenproof, nonstick 23 cm (9 inch) frying pan over a low heat. Add the onion and cook for 6–8 minutes until softened, then stir in the spinach and peas and cook for a further 2 minutes, or until any moisture released by the spinach has evaporated.

2   Beat the eggs in a bowl and season lightly with salt and pepper. Stir in the cooked vegetables, then pour the mixture into the pan and quickly arrange the vegetables so that they are evenly dispersed. Cook over a low heat for 8–10 minutes, or until all but the top of the frittata is set.

3   Transfer the pan to a preheated very hot grill and cook about 10 cm (4 inches) from the heat source until the top is set but not coloured. Give the pan a shake to loosen the frittata, then transfer to a plate to cool.

4   Serve warm or at room temperature, accompanied by a green salad.

Sausage & Sweet Potato Hash

Chicken sausages are a great way to mix things up if you're prone to grabbing the same protein sources across your meals. Sweet potatoes are a source of complex carbohydrates, meaning that the sugars are absorbed more slowly, creating a sustainable energy source – exactly what you need from your PCOS-friendly breakfast!

SERVES **4**

3 tablespoons olive oil

8 chicken sausages

3 large red onions, thinly sliced

500 g (1 lb) sweet potatoes, scrubbed
    and cut into small chunks

8 sage leaves

2 tablespoons balsamic vinegar

salt and pepper

1   Heat the oil in a large frying pan or flameproof casserole and fry the sausages, turning frequently, for about 10 minutes until browned. Transfer the sausages to a plate and set aside.

2   Add the onions to the pan and cook gently, stirring frequently, until lightly browned.

3   Return the sausages to the pan with the sweet potatoes, sage leaves and a little seasoning. Cover the pan with a lid or foil and cook over a very gentle heat for about 25 minutes until the potatoes are tender.

4   Drizzle with the vinegar and check the seasoning before serving.

tip | Feel free to throw in any leftover veggies you have on hand. Dark leafy greens, such as spinach, chard or cavolo nero, make a nice, nutritious addition.

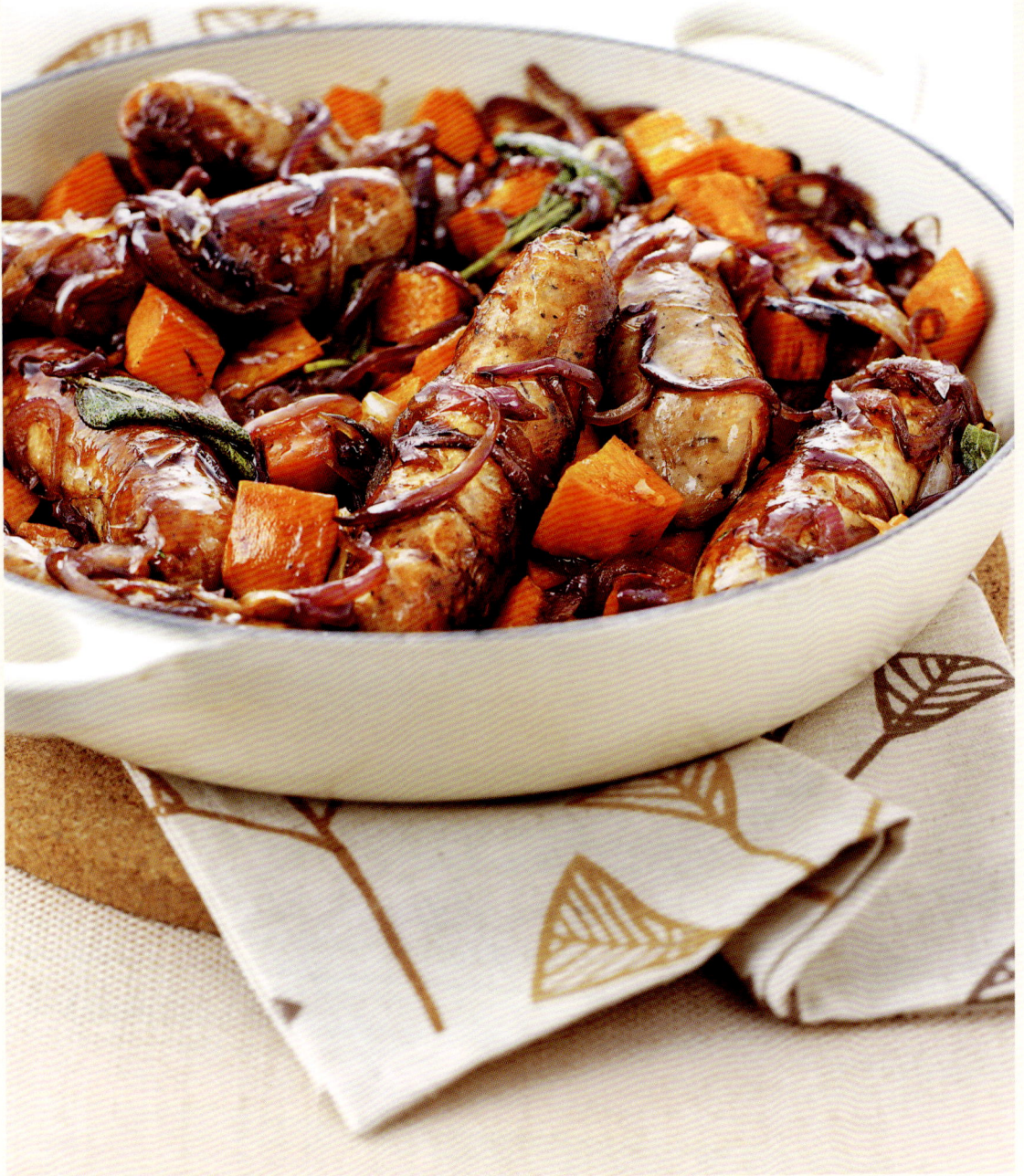

Raspberry & Blueberry Smoothie

Berries are arguably one of the best PCOS staples, great to add to breakfasts, snacks and desserts due to their nutrient density. They are rich in anthocyanins, a phytonutrient that has antioxidant properties, supporting insulin sensitivity, gut health and the cardiovascular system.

SERVES **2**

250 g (8 oz) raspberries
200 ml (7 fl oz) coconut water
200 g (7 oz) blueberries
4 tablespoons Greek yogurt
100 ml (3½ fl oz) coconut milk
1 tablespoon clear honey, or to taste
1 tablespoon milled flaxseed (optional)

1 Purée the raspberries with half of the coconut water.

2 Purée the blueberries with the remaining coconut water.

3 Mix together the yogurt, coconut milk, honey and flaxseed, if using, and add a spoonful of the raspberry purée.

4 Pour the blueberry purée into a tall glass. Carefully pour over the yogurt mixture, and then pour the raspberry purée over the surface of the yogurt. Serve chilled.

tip If you have a protein powder that you love, add a scoop! A high-quality protein powder can be a great staple to keep on hand, ready to boost the protein profile of your smoothies.

Green Smoothie

If you're looking for a breakfast option that is quick, but still ranks high in terms of nutrient density, this green smoothie is for you. It is a delicious way to cram those good-for-you greens in, keeping the fibre high and hitting those anti-inflammatory staples, including ginger and avocado.

SERVES **2**

1 lime, peeled

30 g (1¼ oz) spinach

1 avocado, peeled and stoned

2 celery sticks, plus extra to decorate

1 small thumb-sized piece of ginger

25 g (1 oz) parsley

1 teaspoon green powder (such as
    spirulina, wheatgrass or chlorella)

salt and pepper

1   Juice the lime with the spinach.

2   Transfer the juice to a food processor or blender, add the remaining ingredients and enough water to just cover, then process until smooth. Season the smoothie to taste with salt and pepper, then process again.

3   Pour the smoothie into 2 glasses, add a trimmed celery stick to each glass and serve immediately.

tip | Add a scoop of protein powder for a protein boost.

Snacks,
Light Bites
& Sides

Seeded Oatcakes

These seeded oatcakes make for a super versatile snack and the perfect base for guacamole, nut butter or hummus. Seeds are a nutritious staple to incorporate into your PCOS-friendly diet, as not only do they help to boost the fibre content of your meal or snack with little thought, they also contain a number of beneficial micronutrients, such as vitamin E, zinc and antioxidants.

MAKES **20**

125 g (4 oz) medium oatmeal

75 g (3 oz) plain flour (or substitute with wholemeal flour), plus extra for dusting

4 tablespoons mixed seeds, such as poppy seeds, linseeds and sesame seeds

½ teaspoon celery salt or sea salt flakes

½ teaspoon freshly ground black pepper

50 g (2 oz) unsalted butter, chilled and diced

5 tablespoons cold water

1 Put the oatmeal, flour, seeds, salt and pepper in a bowl or food processor. Add the butter and rub in with the fingertips or process until the mixture resembles breadcrumbs. Add the measured water and mix or blend to a firm dough, adding a little more water if the dough feels dry.

2 Roll out the dough on a lightly floured surface to 2.5 mm (⅛ inch) thick. Cut out 20 rounds using a 6 cm (2½ inch) plain or fluted biscuit cutter, re-rolling the trimmings to make more. Place slightly apart on a large greased baking sheet.

3 Bake in a preheated oven, 180°C (350°F), Gas Mark 4, for about 25 minutes until firm.

4 Transfer to a wire rack to cool. Serve with guacamole (see page 77).

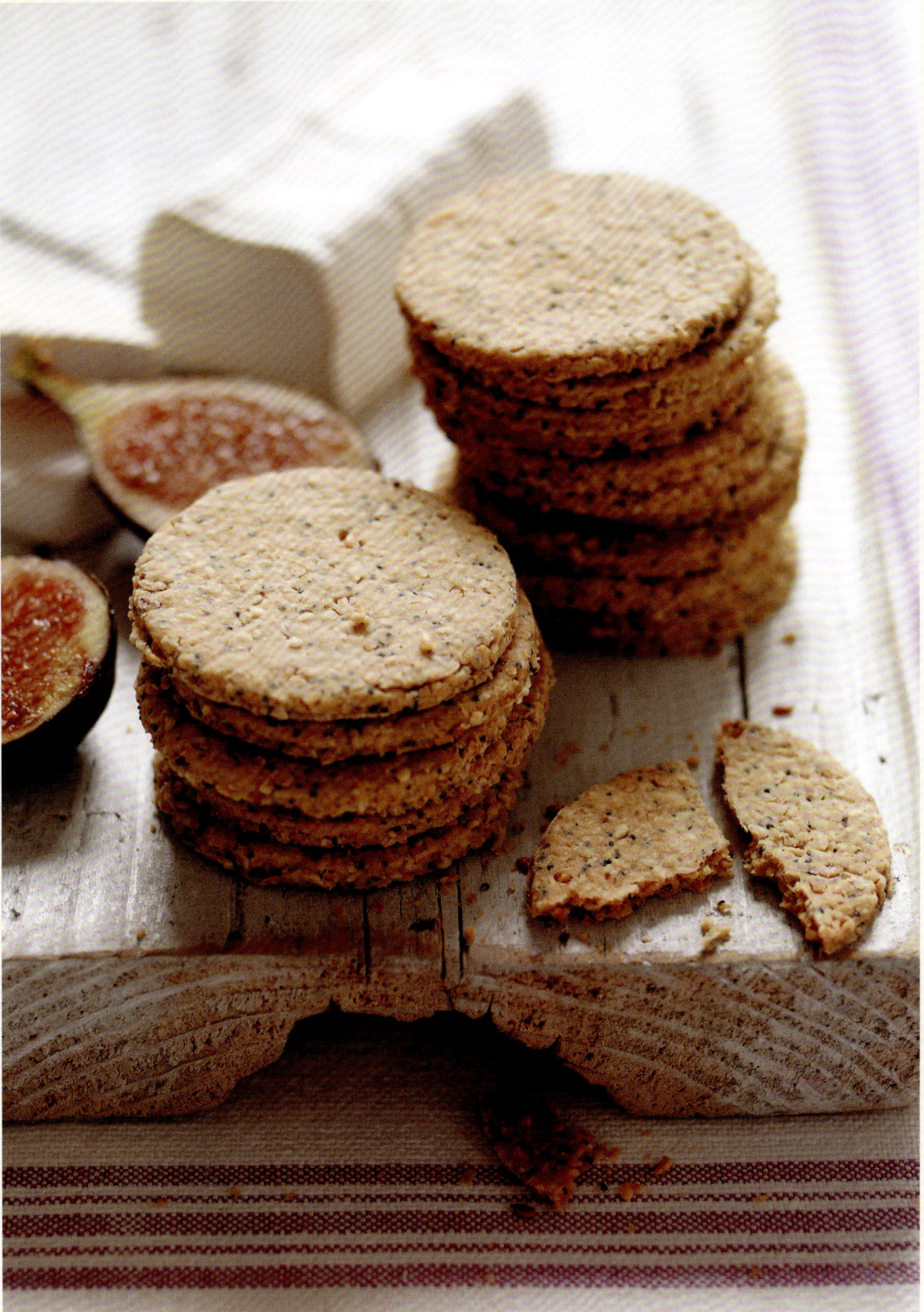

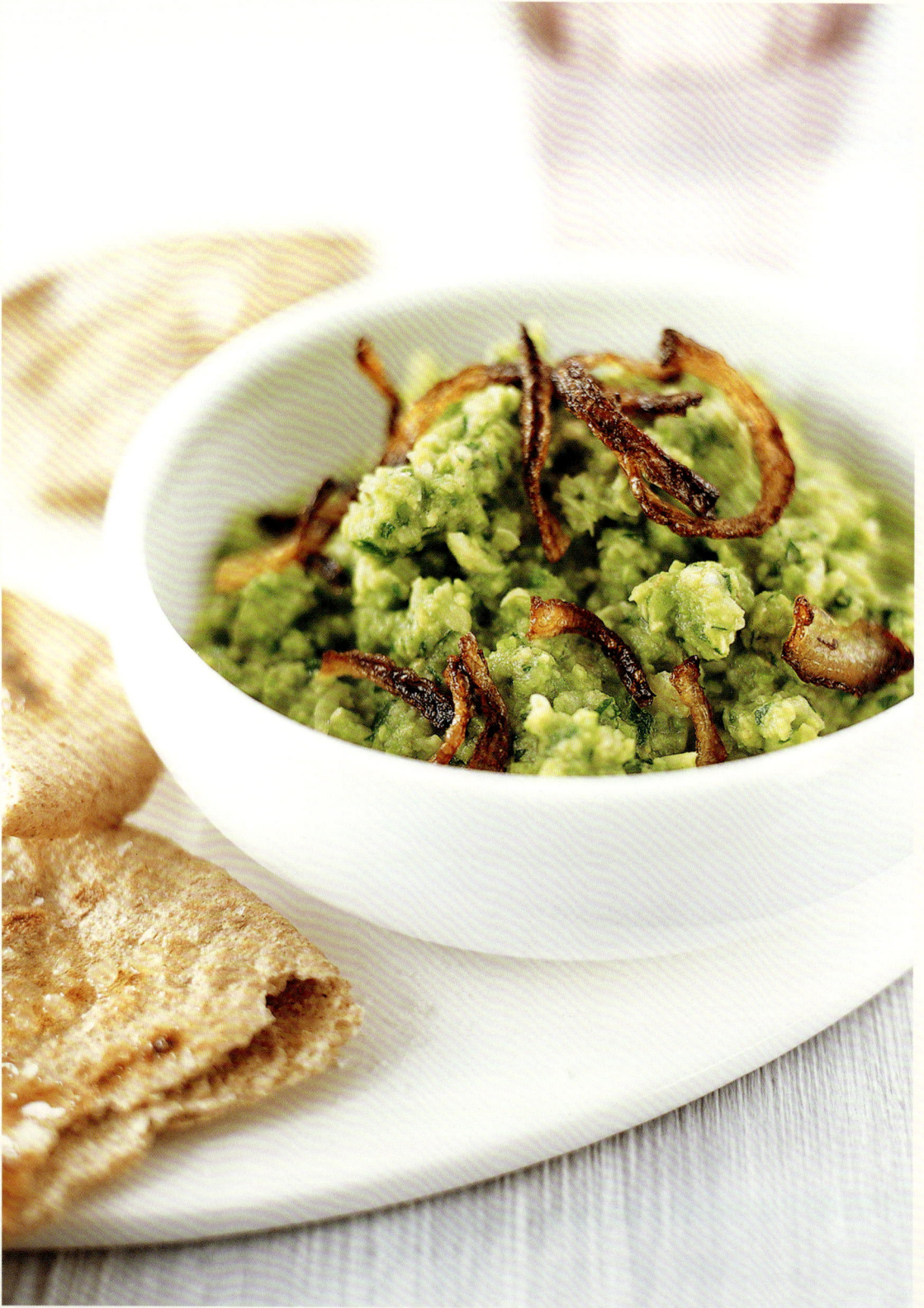

Broad Bean & Chilli Dip

If you haven't tried broad beans, they aren't too dissimilar in taste and texture to edamame beans. They make a great dip when blended, and contain a good amount of fibre and protein, making them a great PCOS-friendly snack.

SERVES **4**

375 g (12 oz) fresh or frozen broad beans
50 g (2 oz) flat leaf parsley, coarsely chopped
50 g (2 oz) coriander, coarsely chopped
1–2 mild green chillies, deseeded
    and chopped
2 garlic cloves, chopped
1½ teaspoons ground cumin
3 tablespoons olive oil
1 onion, thinly sliced
salt

1   Cook the beans in a pan of salted boiling water for 5 minutes. Add the herbs, cover and simmer for a further 5 minutes. Drain, reserving some of the cooking liquid.

2   Place the cooked beans and herbs in a blender or food processor with the chillies, garlic, cumin, 2 tablespoons of the oil and 3–4 tablespoons of the reserved cooking liquid. Process to a smooth paste. Season to taste and add a little more cooking liquid if it is too dry. Transfer to a serving dish and chill until required.

3   When ready to serve, heat the remaining oil in a nonstick frying pan and fry the onion briskly until golden and crisp. Scatter the crispy onions over the dip and serve.

Cheese & Spinach Quesadillas

Being overprepared with your snacks is a great way to make sure you're never caught out. If you're prone to letting hunger take over, grabbing the first sweet thing you see as a pick-me-up, you might find that you're constantly craving sugar and a quick hit of energy. By having a protein-rich snack instead, it can help break that cycle. You can prep these quesadillas ahead of time, ready to combat hunger and prevent grazing.

SERVES 4

275 g (9 oz) baby spinach leaves

8 wholemeal tortillas

250 g (8 oz) goats' cheese

2 tablespoons sun-dried tomatoes, chopped

2 avocados, peeled, stoned and diced

1 red onion, thinly sliced

juice of 1 lime

2 tablespoons chopped coriander

salt and pepper

1 Place the spinach in a pan with a small amount of water, then cover and cook until wilted. Drain and squeeze dry.

2 Heat 2 nonstick frying pans over a medium heat. Add 1 tortilla to each and crumble a quarter of the goats' cheese, followed by a quarter of the spinach and sun-dried tomatoes, over each tortilla. Season well. Place another tortilla on top of each one and cook for 3–4 minutes until golden underneath.

3 Gently turn the quesadillas over and cook for a further 3–4 minutes. Remove from the pans and keep warm.

4 Repeat steps 2 and 3 with the remaining tortillas.

5 Meanwhile, mix together the avocados, onion, lime juice and coriander in a bowl.

6 Serve the quesadillas in wedges with the avocado salsa on the side.

tip There is no limit to what vegetables you can pop in your quesadillas. They can also double up as an easy, meal-prepped lunch option.

Boiled Egg
with Mustard Soldiers

Eggs are small in size, but that doesn't mean that they don't have big health benefits. When it comes to including a healthy amount of micronutrients for PCOS, eggs are a really easy way to hit your goals. They are rich in choline for brain health, vitamins A and D which support fertility, and B12 for energy production. Egg recipes don't have to be over-complicated, and this one is a great example of a simple yet delicious way to pack in those micronutrients.

SERVES 4

2 teaspoons wholegrain mustard, or to taste
50 g (2 oz) unsalted butter, softened
4 large eggs
4 thick slices of sourdough bread
black pepper
mustard greens and cress, to serve

1   Beat the mustard, butter and some pepper together in a small bowl.

2   Cook the eggs in a saucepan of boiling water for 4–5 minutes until softly set.

3   Meanwhile, toast the bread, then butter one side with the mustard butter. Cut into fingers.

4   Serve the eggs with the mustard soldiers, with mustard greens and cress on the side.

tip | You can also dunk vegetables, such as steamed Tenderstem broccoli, roasted courgettes or peppers, into your egg – there are no limits!

Minted Pea & Sesame Falafel

Homemade falafel are a great way to increase your fibre intake. Chickpeas form the base, but there are no limits on the other types of vegetables, herbs and spices you can add to the mix. Here, peas and mint add a lovely freshness to the creamy chickpeas. They make a great on-the-go snack.

SERVES **4**

250 g (8 oz) frozen peas, just defrosted

2 x 400 g (13 oz) cans chickpeas, drained

1 onion, peeled and quartered

1½ teaspoons cumin seeds, roughly crushed

1½ teaspoons coriander seeds, roughly crushed

1 teaspoon ground turmeric

3 tablespoons chopped mint

2 tablespoons sesame seeds

1 tablespoon plain flour

3 tablespoons olive oil

salt and pepper

RADISH CACIK

200 g (7 oz) low-fat natural yogurt

100 g (3½ oz) radishes, finely diced

5-cm (2-inch) piece of cucumber, finely diced

2 tablespoons chopped mint

1   Finely chop the peas, chickpeas and onion together in a blender or food processor. Alternatively, chop them finely with a knife. Mix in the crushed seeds, turmeric and mint. Season with salt and pepper.

2   Spoon 20 mounds of the mixture on to a baking sheet, then roll into ovals with the palms of your hands. Mix the sesame seeds and flour on a plate, then roll the falafel in the mixture and return to the baking sheet. Cover and chill until required.

3   Mix all the cacik ingredients together, season to taste and spoon into a serving bowl. Cover and chill until required.

4   When ready to serve, heat 2 tablespoons of the oil in a large frying pan, add the falafel and fry, turning, until golden brown and piping hot, adding the remaining oil if needed.

5   Serve immediately with the cacik, a green salad and warmed pitta breads.

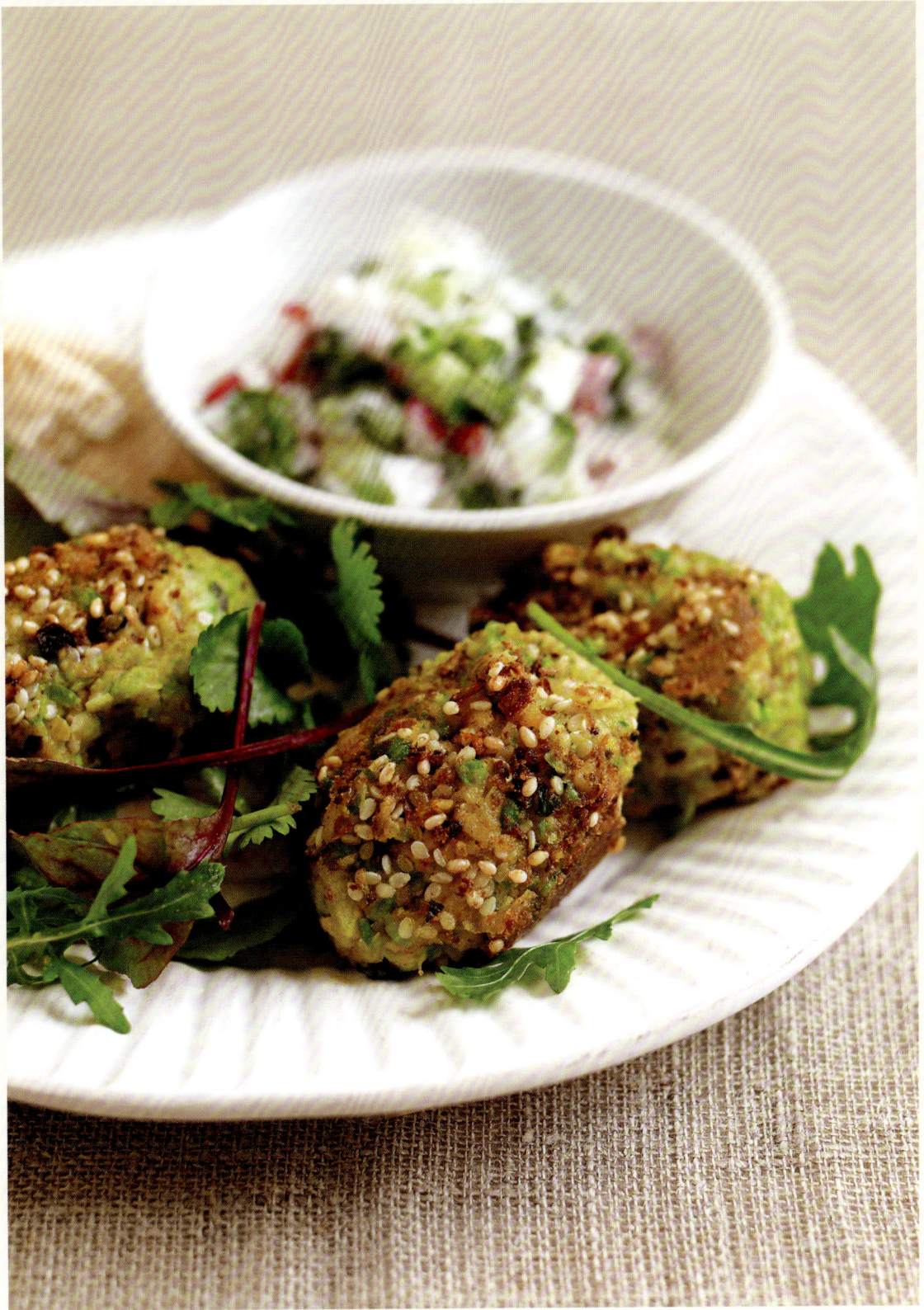

Crunchy Pesto Broccoli
with Poached Eggs

You can't go wrong pairing eggs and veg. This quick, nutritious lunch makes getting in those nutrient-dense greens effortless. The combination of the healthy fats from the pesto, fibre from the veggies and protein in the eggs will keep your blood sugar levels stable across the rest of the afternoon, preventing any dips or sugar cravings.

SERVES 4

625 g (1¼ lb) broccoli florets
300 g (10 oz) sugar snap peas
4 eggs
75 g (3 oz) sun-dried tomatoes, chopped
pepper
Parmesan cheese shavings, to serve

PESTO

10 g (⅓ oz) basil leaves
5 g (¼ oz) toasted pine nuts
5 g (¼ oz) Parmesan cheese, grated
1 small garlic clove, crushed
15–20 ml (½– ¾ fl oz) olive oil

tip | For more protein, up the egg count!

1   To make the pesto, place the basil and pine nuts in a food processor and blitz until broken down. Add the cheese and garlic and blitz briefly. With the motor still running, slowly pour in the oil through the feed tube until combined.

2   Cook the broccoli and sugar snap peas in a large saucepan of boiling water for 7–8 minutes until 'al dente'.

3   Meanwhile, bring a saucepan of water to a gentle simmer and stir with a large spoon to create a swirl. Break 2 of the eggs into the water and cook for 3 minutes. Remove with a slotted spoon and keep warm. Repeat with the remaining eggs.

4   Drain the vegetables, then return them to the pan and add 1½ tablespoons of the pesto (store any remaining pesto in an airtight container in the refrigerator) and the sun-dried tomatoes. Gently toss together until well coated.

5   Serve topped with the poached eggs and Parmesan shavings and sprinkled with pepper.

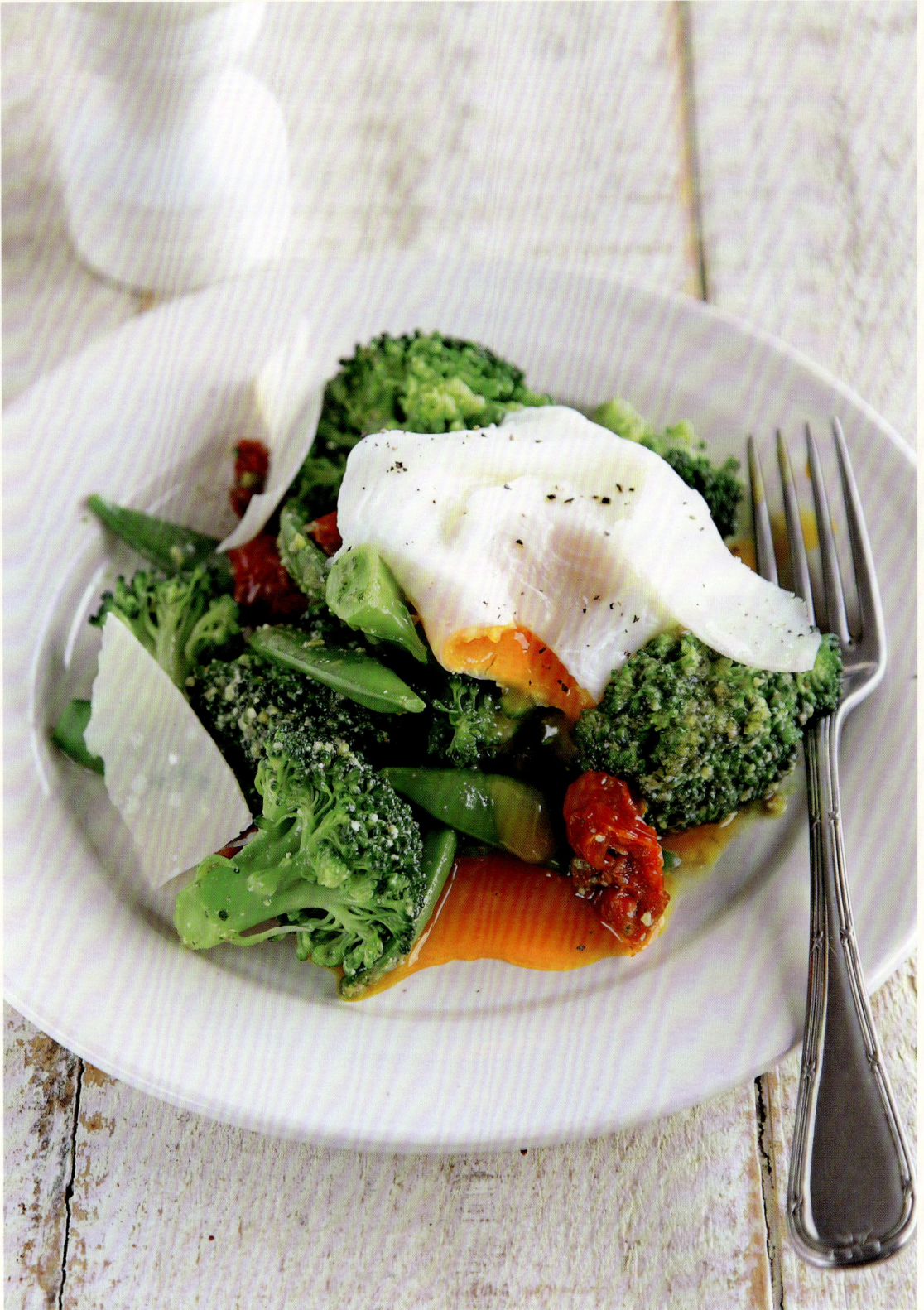

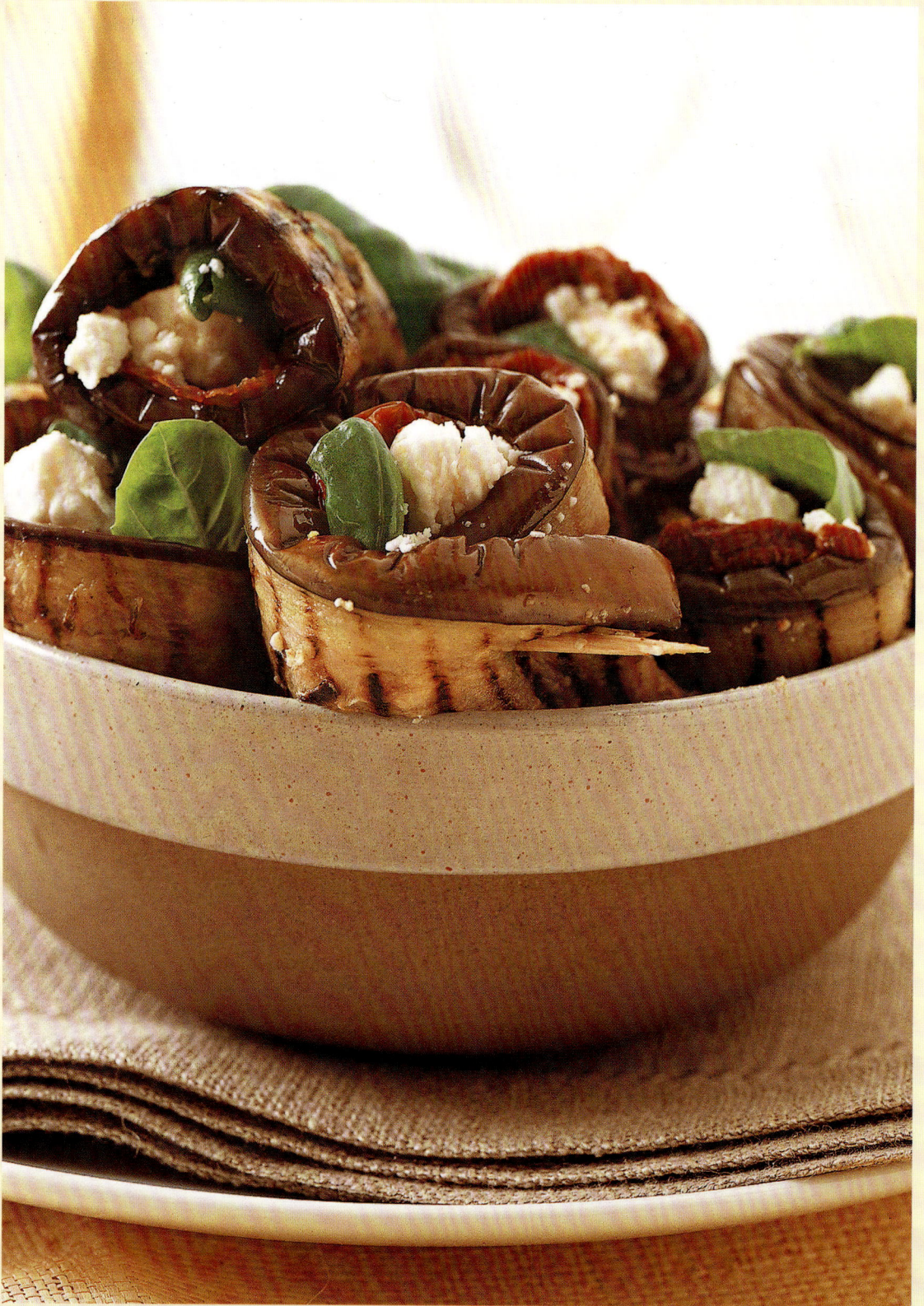

Aubergine, Tomato & Feta Rolls

If you're a roasted veggie fan, you'll love these aubergine, tomato and feta rolls. They are a great PCOS snack option as they are low in carbs but contain a good amount of fibre from the vegetables. Plus, feta is a great vegetarian protein source. You can also play around with the combinations here.

SERVES **4**

2 aubergines

3 tablespoons olive oil

125 g (4 oz) feta cheese, roughly diced

12 sun-dried tomatoes in oil, drained

15–20 basil leaves

salt and pepper

1   Trim the ends of the aubergines, then cut a thin slice lengthways from either side of each; discard these slices, which should be mainly skin. Cut each aubergine lengthways into 4 slices.

2   Heat the grill on the hottest setting or heat a griddle pan until very hot.

3   Brush both sides of the aubergine slices with the oil, then cook under the grill or in the griddle pan for 3 minutes on each side, or until browned and softened.

4   Lay the aubergine slices on a board and divide the feta, tomatoes and basil leaves between them. Season well with salt and pepper. Roll up each slice from a short end and secure with a cocktail stick. Arrange on serving plates and serve immediately, or cover and set aside in a cool place (not the refrigerator) and serve at room temperature when required.

Moroccan-spiced Chickpeas

If you've never made crispy chickpeas, you're in for a treat! They take on a whole new texture, not too dissimilar to nuts, making for a great snack option if you love a bit of crunch. Chickpeas are rich in vitamin B6, promoting a stable mood and nervous system.

SERVES **4**

2 x 400 g (13 oz) cans chickpeas, drained
   and rinsed
1 tablespoon olive oil
1 tablespoon rose harissa paste
1 tablespoon Moroccan or Middle
   Eastern spice mix, such as baharat
½ teaspoon salt

1 Dry the chickpeas on kitchen paper to remove any excess water.

2 Mix all the remaining ingredients together in a large bowl. Add the chickpeas and toss in the spice mix to coat.

3 Spread the chickpeas out in a single layer on a rimmed baking sheet and roast in a preheated oven, 200°C (400°F), Gas Mark 6, for 35–40 minutes until a deep golden colour. Leave to cool before serving.

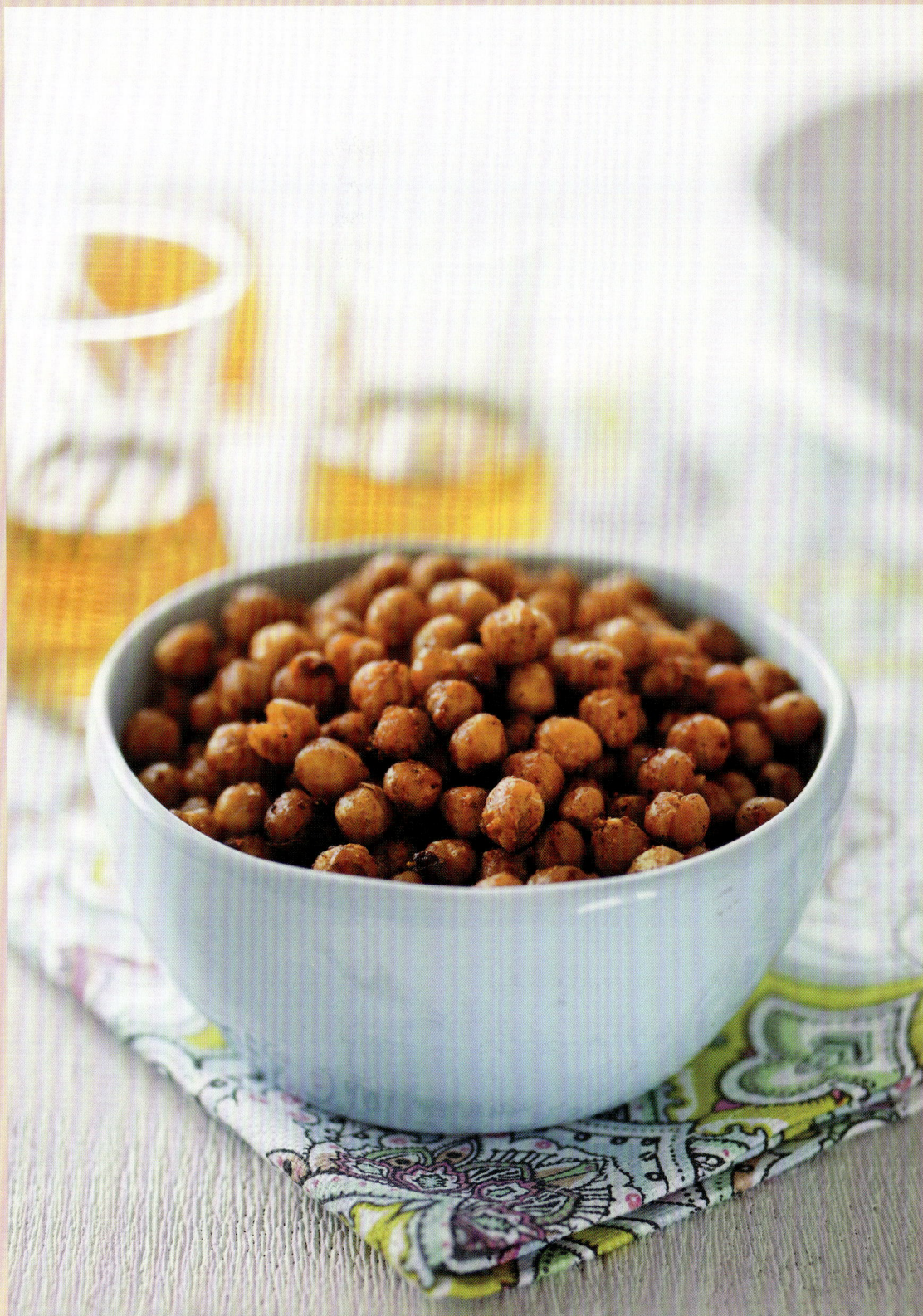

Chicken Dippers
with Hummus

By including protein, fat and carbohydrates in your snack, your blood sugar levels remain stable rather than spiking, as they can do with carbohydrate-dense options. In this recipe, chicken is your protein source while hummus contains carbohydrates from chickpeas, and healthy fats in the form of tahini.

SERVES **4**

1 tablespoon almond flour
1 tablespoon chopped parsley
1 tablespoon chopped coriander
300 g (10 oz) chicken mini-fillets
25 g (1 oz) butter
1 tablespoon olive oil

HUMMUS

1 garlic clove, finely diced
400 g (13 oz) can chickpeas, rinsed
    and drained
juice of ½ lemon
2 tablespoons tahini paste
3–4 tablespoons extra virgin olive oil

1   Mix together the flour and herbs on a plate, then toss the chicken strips in the herbed flour.

2   Heat the butter and olive oil in a large frying pan, add the chicken and cook for 3–4 minutes on each side, or until golden and cooked through.

3   Meanwhile, make the hummus. Place the garlic, chickpeas, lemon juice and tahini in a food processor or blender and blend until nearly smooth. With the motor still running, pour in the extra virgin olive oil through the feed tube and blend to the desired consistency.

4   Serve the chicken with the hummus for dipping.

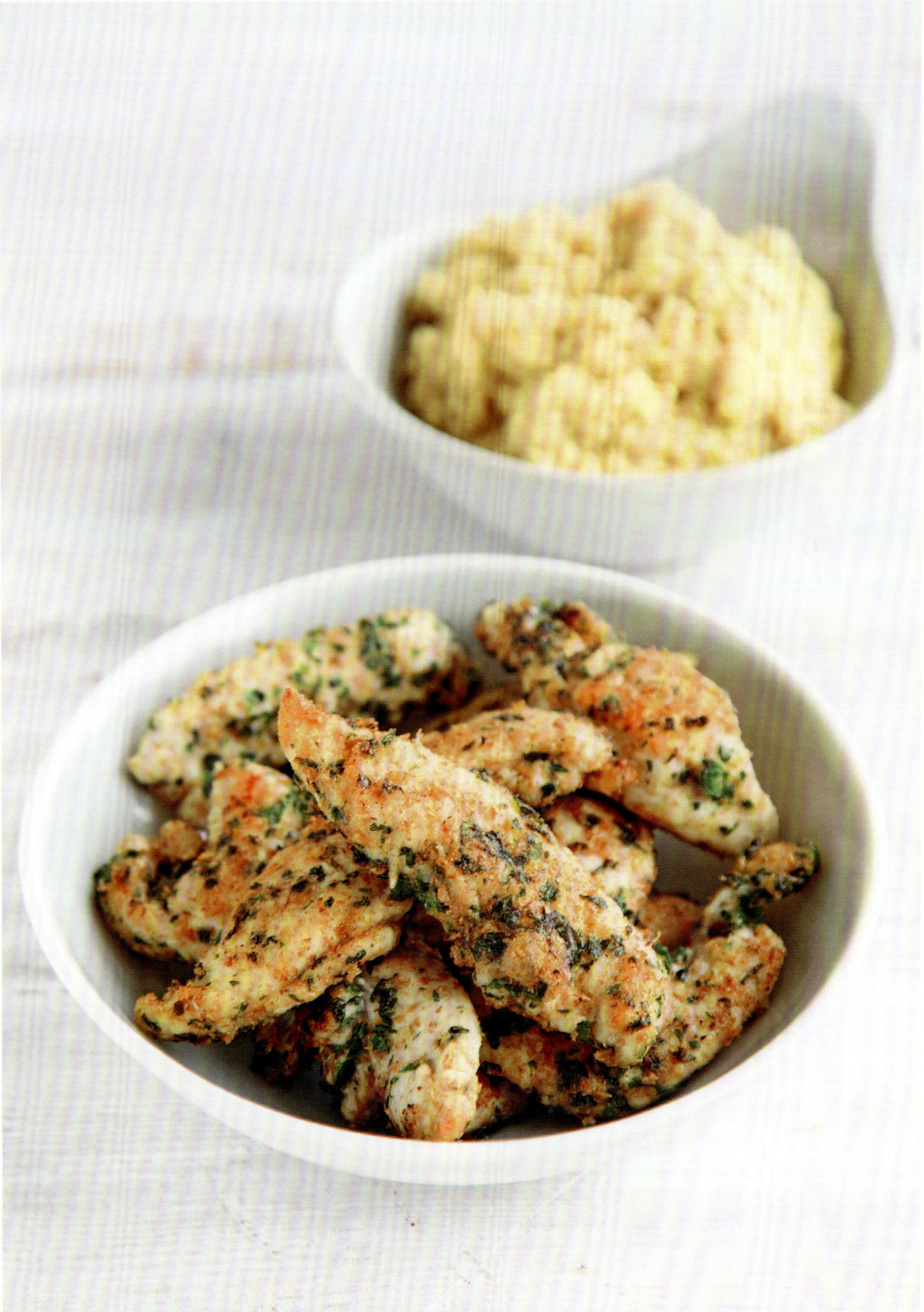

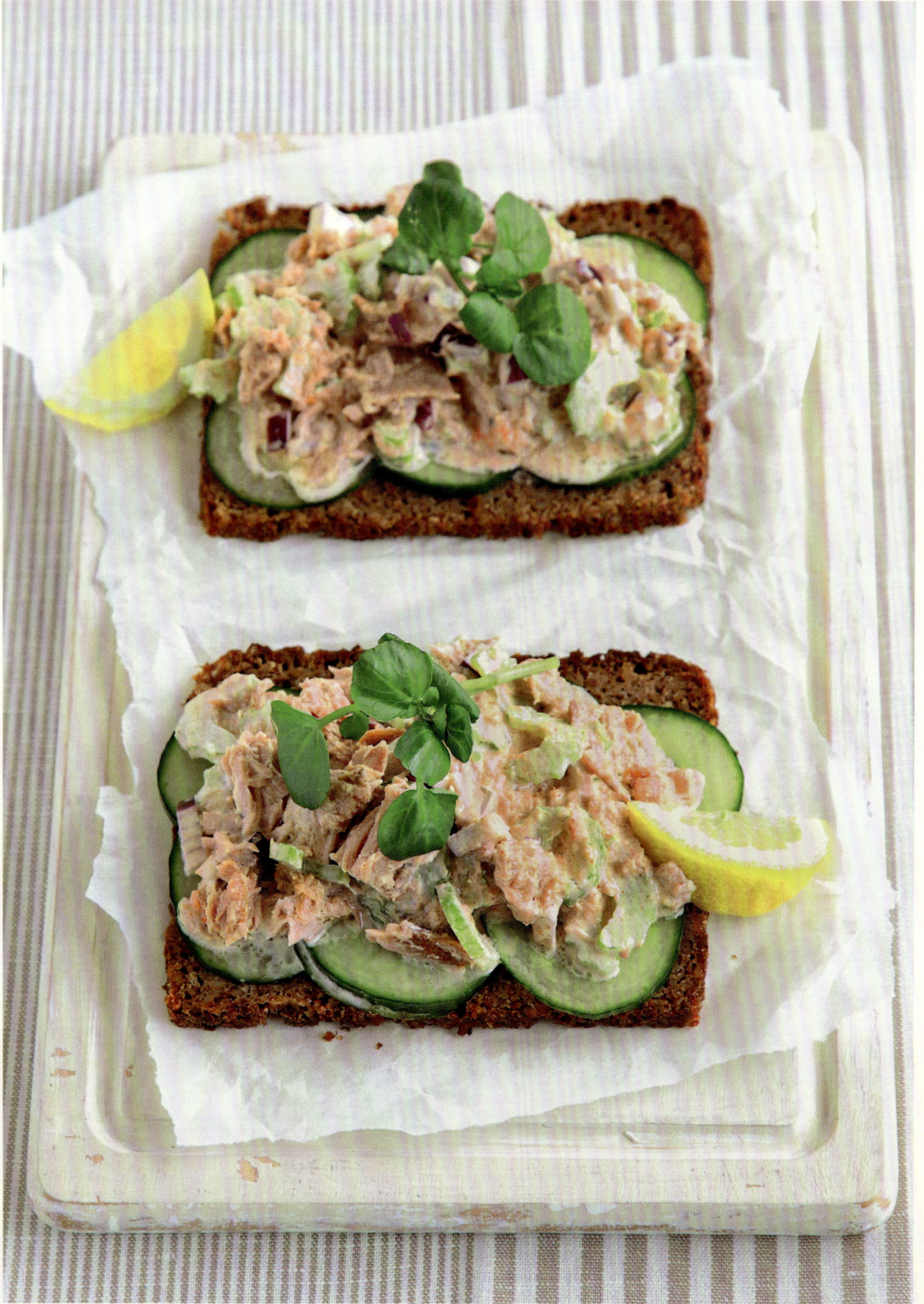

Spiced Tuna Open Sandwiches

High-fibre bread such as pumpernickel, a type of rye, is a great staple to keep on hand for quick snacks or lunches. These types of loaves are higher in fibre than conventional white bread and contain a number of beneficial micronutrients, such as B vitamins and selenium, which are also found in tuna. Pumpernickel also contains lignans, a compound found in some plants that has antioxidant properties and may help to regulate oestrogen activity in the body.

SERVES **4**

2 x 250 g (8 oz) cans tuna, drained
4 tablespoons natural yogurt
2 tablespoons thinly sliced celery
¼ teaspoon smoked paprika
¼ teaspoon cayenne pepper
1 tablespoon finely chopped red onion
juice of ½ lemon
¼ cucumber, thinly sliced
4 slices of pumpernickel bread
a few sprigs of watercress, to garnish
lemon wedges, to serve

1   Flake the tuna in a bowl, then mix together with the yogurt, celery, paprika, cayenne pepper, onion and lemon juice.

2   Arrange the slices of cucumber on the pumpernickel, then top with the tuna mixture.

3   Garnish with a few sprigs of watercress and serve with lemon wedges.

Prawn & Spinach Scrambled Eggs

This recipe is low-carb and high in protein, making it a great PCOS-friendly snack or quick lunch. It'll keep you full and satisfied, and blood sugar levels stable. Eggs contain good amounts of choline, which supports brain health, while prawns are rich in zinc which can help to regulate androgen levels.

SERVES **4**

1 tablespoon olive oil

150 g (5 oz) small raw peeled prawns

75 g (3 oz) spinach leaves

4 eggs

1 egg yolk

25 g (1 oz) butter, cubed

salt and pepper

pinch of hot smoked paprika, to serve

1   Heat the oil in a frying pan, add the prawns and cook for 3 minutes, turning once, until they turn pink and are cooked through. Remove from the pan and set aside.

2   Place the spinach in a large colander and pour over boiling water until wilted. Leave to cool slightly, then squeeze out any excess water.

3   Break the eggs into the pan and add the egg yolk, then season and scatter over the butter. Cook over a low heat for a couple of minutes until the whites begin to set.

4   Stir in the spinach and prawns, gently breaking up the yolks. Cook for a further 1–2 minutes until the egg is just set and the prawns are piping hot. Serve sprinkled with a little paprika.

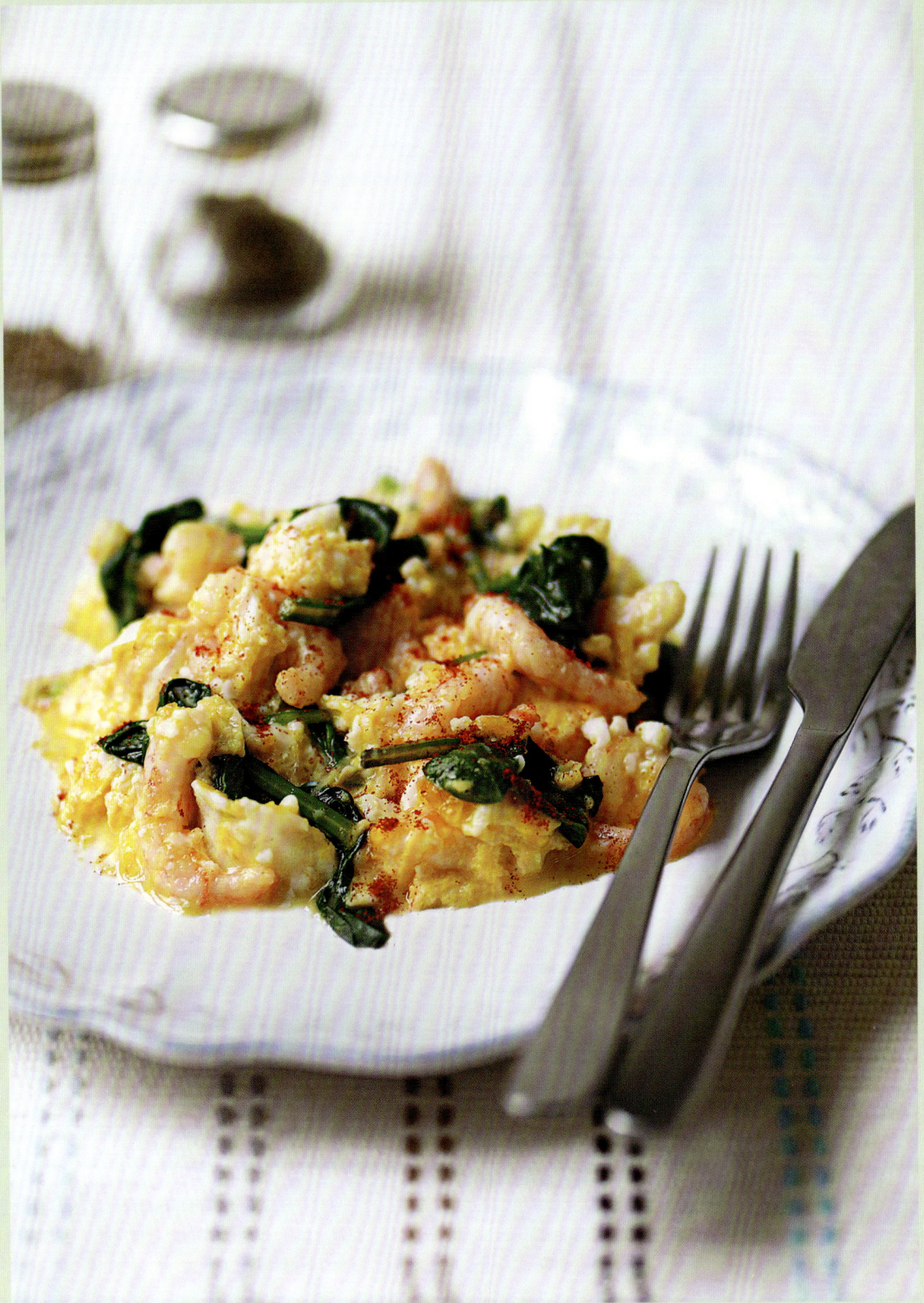

SNACKS, LIGHT BITES & SIDES

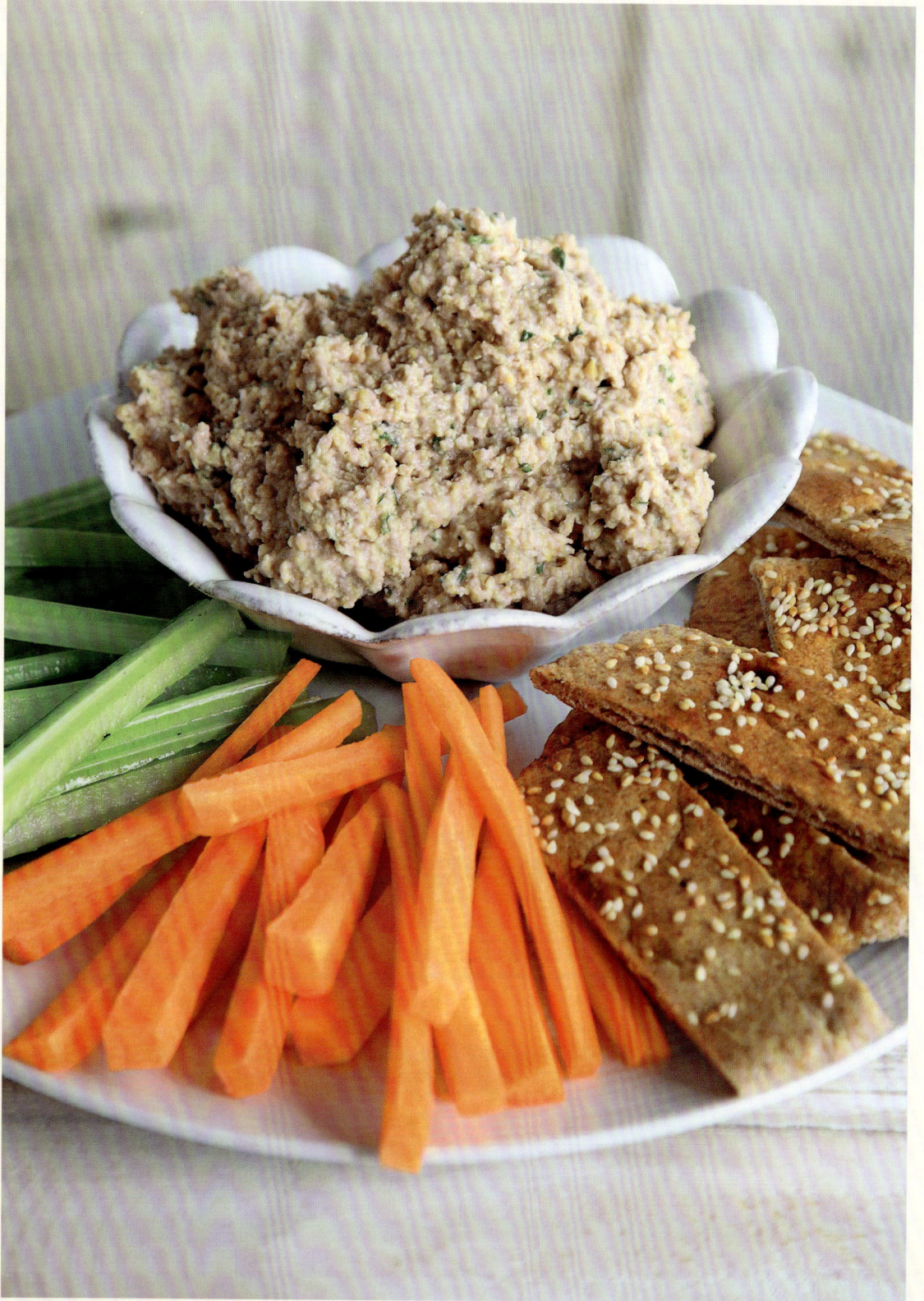

Walnut Hummus
with Carrot & Celery Sticks

You can't get more classic than hummus and veggies for a nutritious snack option. Hummus contains all three macronutrients – complex carbohydrates, protein and fat – plus a number of PCOS-supportive micronutrients. The high fibre content of chickpeas alongside vegetables to dip helps to keep your blood sugar levels stable, banishing mid-afternoon dips and cravings.

SERVES 4

4 tablespoons extra virgin olive oil,
    plus extra for brushing
2 garlic cloves, crushed
40 g (1¾ oz) walnuts
400 g (13 oz) can chickpeas, rinsed
    and drained
1½ tablespoons tahini paste
juice of ½ lemon
½ tablespoon chopped coriander
salt and pepper

TO SERVE

2 wholemeal pitta breads
2 tablespoons sesame seeds
2 large carrots, peeled and cut
    into batons
4 celery sticks, cut into batons

1   Heat the oil in a frying pan, add the garlic and cook for 2–3 minutes. Remove from the heat and leave to cool slightly.

2   Heat a nonstick frying pan over a medium-low heat and dry-fry the walnuts for 3–4 minutes, stirring frequently, until slightly golden and giving off an aroma.

3   Place the chickpeas, tahini, lemon juice, garlic oil and toasted walnuts in a food processor and process until smooth, adding a little water to loosen the mixture if necessary. Stir in the coriander and season to taste. Spoon into a bowl.

4   Toast the pitta breads under a preheated medium grill for 4 minutes, then turn over, brush with oil and sprinkle with the sesame seeds. Toast until golden, then cut into strips.

5   Serve the hummus with the pitta strips and the carrot and celery sticks.

Mixed Seed Soda Bread

There is nothing quite like the feeling of baking your own bread! Opting for wholemeal flour and including fibrous extras like seeds is a great way to up the fibre profile to create a PCOS-friendly loaf. Top with healthy fats and a source of protein, such as hummus, or dunk in a hearty stew.

MAKES **1 SMALL LOAF**

spray oil, for oiling

350 g (11½ oz) wholemeal plain flour,
     plus extra for dusting and sprinkling

50 g (2 oz) sunflower seeds

2 tablespoons poppy seeds

1 teaspoon bicarbonate of soda

1 teaspoon salt

1 teaspoon caster sugar

300 ml (½ pint) buttermilk

1 Lightly oil a baking sheet with spray oil. Mix the flour, sunflower seeds, poppy seeds, bicarbonate of soda, salt and sugar together in a bowl. Make a well in the centre, add the buttermilk and gradually work into the flour mixture to form a soft dough.

2 Turn the dough out on to a lightly floured work surface and knead for 5 minutes. Shape into a flattish round. Transfer to the prepared baking sheet. Using a sharp knife, cut a cross in the top of the bread. Sprinkle a little extra flour over the surface.

3 Bake in a preheated oven, 230°C (450°F), Gas Mark 8, for 15 minutes, then reduce the temperature to 200°C (400°F), Gas Mark 6, and bake for a further 25–30 minutes until risen and the loaf sounds hollow when tapped underneath. Leave to cool completely on a wire rack.

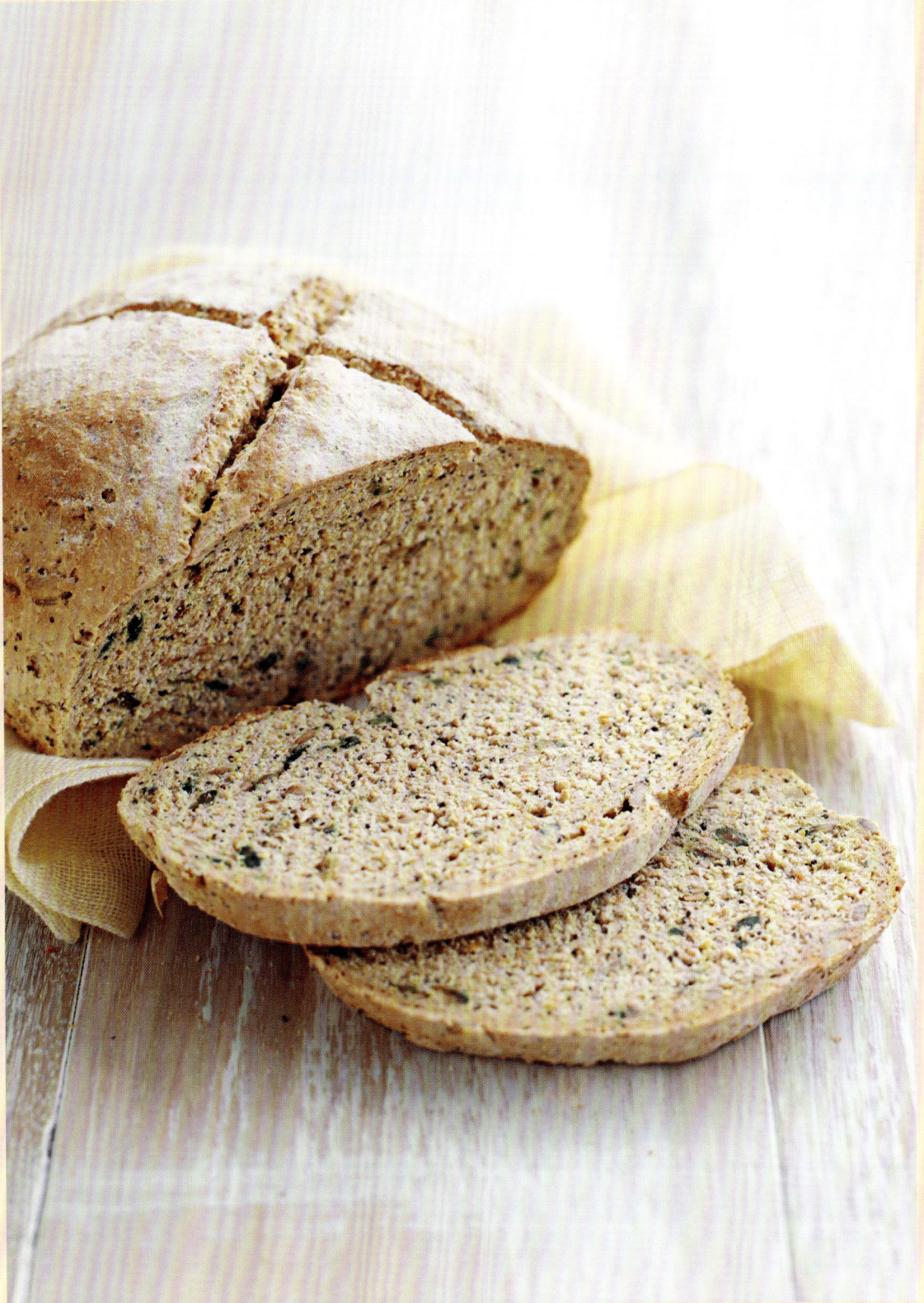

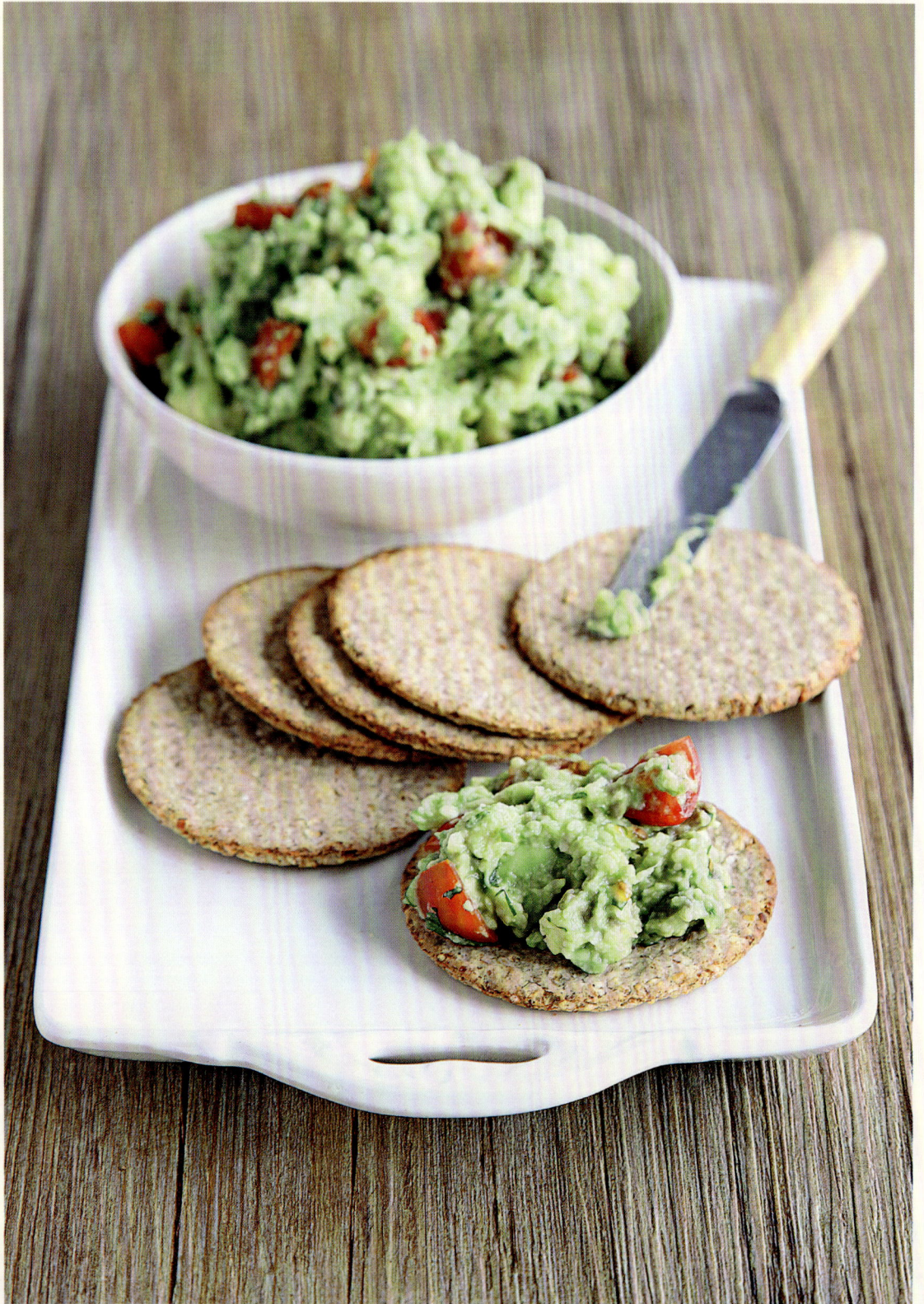

Guacamole

Guacamole makes for the perfect PCOS-friendly snack. Avocado is rich in fibre and monounsaturated fat, both of which contribute to a healthy cardiovascular system and improve cholesterol status, a key consideration for those with PCOS. It also contains vitamins C and E, which have antioxidant properties, supporting healthy, glowing skin. What's more, it takes a matter of minutes to whip up, making it a great snack when you're short on time.

SERVES 4

2 ripe avocados, peeled, stoned
   and chopped
juice of 1 lime
6 cherry tomatoes, diced
1 tablespoon chopped coriander
1–2 garlic cloves, crushed
oatcakes or vegetable crudités, to serve

1 Put the avocados and lime juice in a bowl and immediately mash together to prevent discoloration, then stir in the remaining ingredients.

2 Serve immediately with oatcakes or vegetable crudités.

tip This guacamole goes well with the Turkey Burgers with Sweet Potato Wedges (*see* page 168) or with the Seeded Oatcakes (*see* page 52).

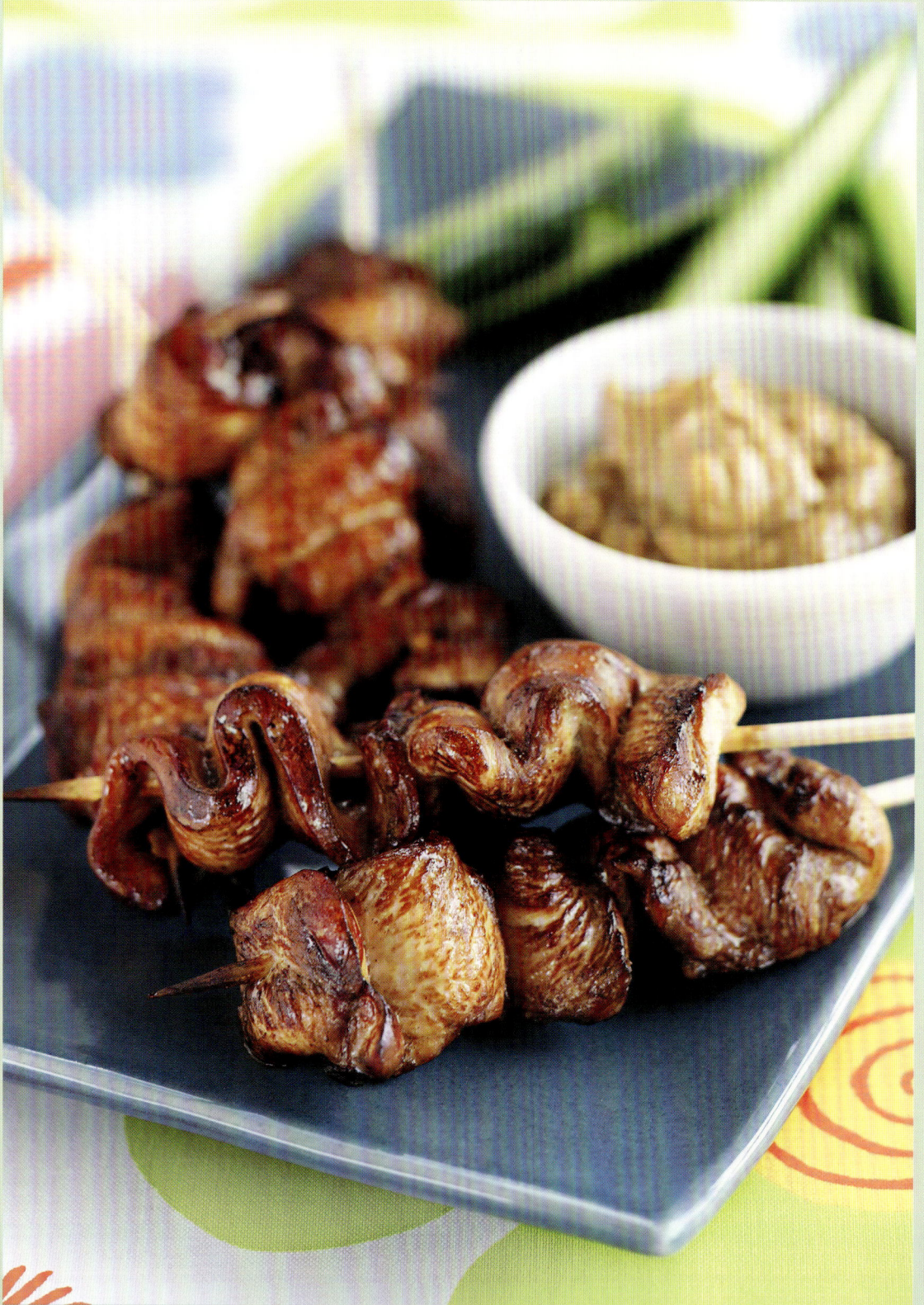

Chicken Satay Skewers

Moving away from conventional snack foods, such as cereal bars and crisps, can help make a positive impact on both how you feel across the day and PCOS symptoms. Many typical choices are high in refined sugars and low in protein, dysregulating blood sugar levels and the hormone insulin. Instead, opting for high-protein snacks like these chicken satay skewers will help to regulate insulin and manage the symptoms of PCOS.

SERVES 4

6 tablespoons dark soy sauce
2 tablespoons sesame oil
1 teaspoon Chinese 5-spice powder
375 g (12 oz) boneless, skinless chicken
    breasts, cut into long, thin strips

SAUCE

4 tablespoons peanut butter or
    almond butter
1 tablespoon dark soy sauce
½ teaspoon ground coriander
½ teaspoon ground cumin
pinch of paprika or chilli powder
8 tablespoons water
cucumber, cut into strips, to serve

1   Place the soy sauce, sesame oil and 5-spice powder into a bowl and mix. Add the chicken and toss together to coat in the marinade. Cover and set aside for 1 hour, stirring occasionally.

2   Thread the chicken, in a zigzag fashion, on to 10 soaked bamboo skewers (soaking them in warm water for 30 minutes will prevent the sticks burning while cooking), and place the chicken under a preheated hot grill for 8–10 minutes, turning once, until golden and cooked through.

3   Meanwhile, put all the sauce ingredients in a small pan and heat, stirring, until warm and well mixed. Transfer to a small serving bowl.

4   Place the bowl of sauce on a serving plate with the cucumber on one side and the hot chicken skewers around it.

Spicy Tuna Skewers

If you're not quite sure about how to include anti-inflammatory spices like turmeric and ginger in your diet, incorporating them into a marinade for your protein source couldn't be more straightforward. These tuna skewers are a great example of how you can achieve this, reaping the health benefits of these spices, all while giving your fish a bit of added oomph!

SERVES **4**

1 tablespoon ground turmeric

1 tablespoon ground cumin

1 tablespoon ground coriander

3.5-cm (1½-inch) piece of fresh root
  ginger, peeled and finely chopped

2 tablespoons olive oil

2 garlic cloves, crushed

400 g (13 oz) fresh tuna steak, cut
  into chunks

200 ml (7 fl oz) natural yogurt

finely grated zest of 1 lemon

vegetable oil, for brushing

salt and pepper

1 Put the turmeric, cumin, coriander, ginger, olive oil and 1 of the garlic cloves in a bowl and stir well. Add the tuna, coating all the pieces with the mix. Cover and leave in the refrigerator to marinate for at least 1 hour, preferably overnight.

2 Mix the yogurt with the remaining garlic clove and the lemon zest and season with salt and pepper.

3 Heat a griddle pan over a high heat and brush with a little vegetable oil. Sear the tuna pieces in batches for 1 minute on 1 side and 30 seconds on the other. Remove from the pan and serve with bamboo skewers for dipping into the yogurt sauce.

tip Salmon or any other firm protein source, such as tofu, tempeh or even chicken, also works well here.

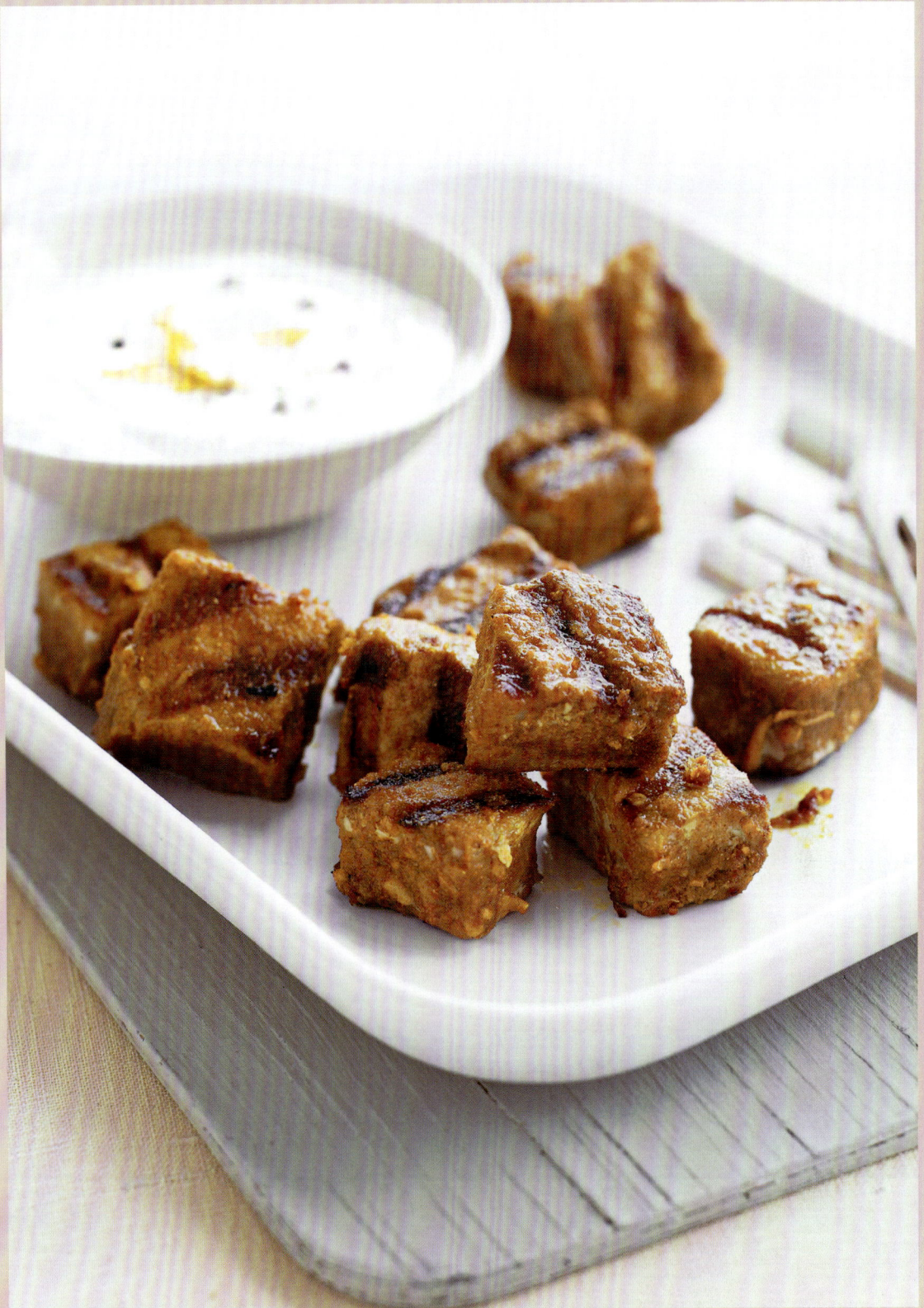

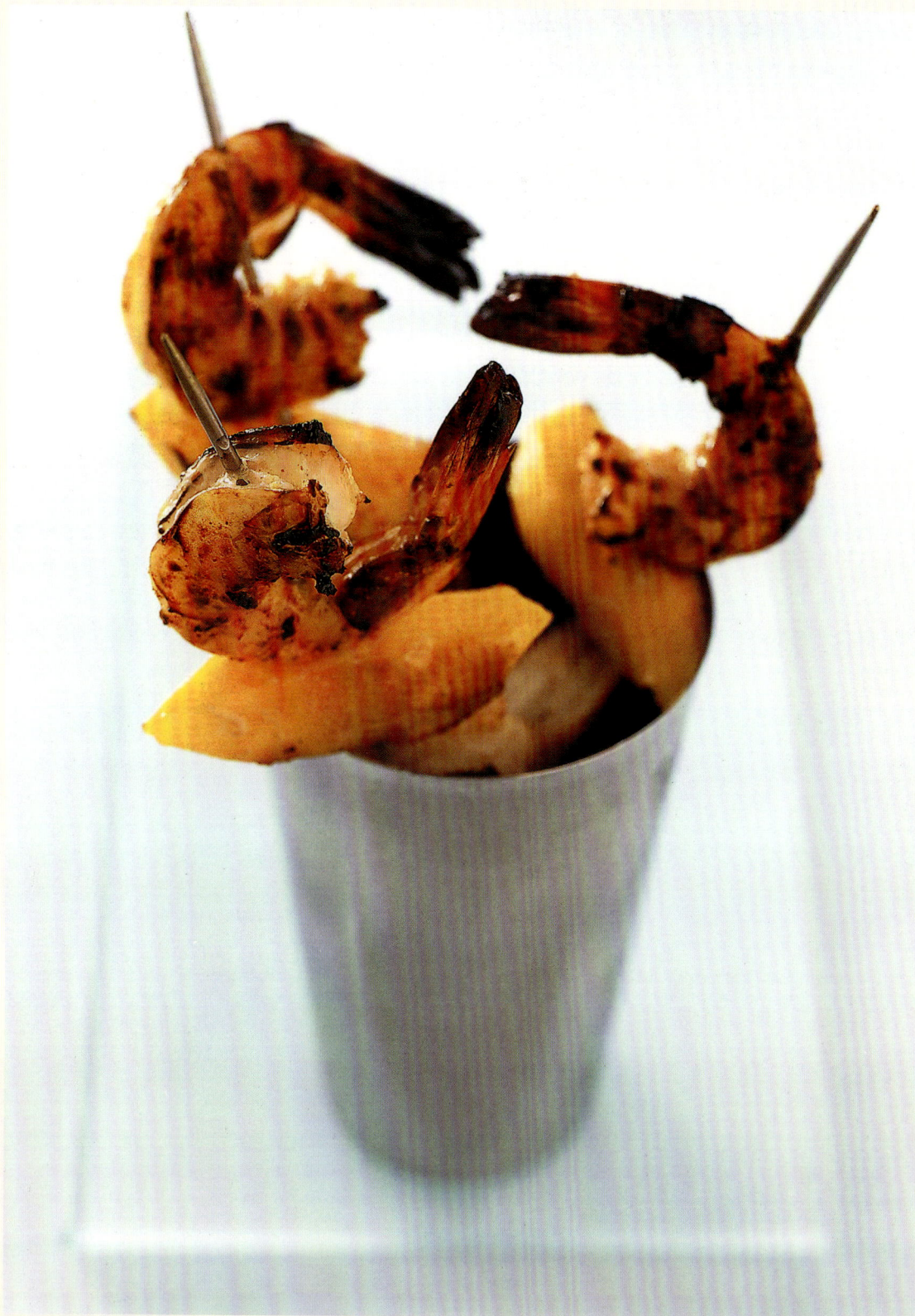

Prawn & Mango Kebabs

There is a bit of noise around avoiding tropical fruits if you have PCOS due to their higher sugar content, but in reality, you can still include them in your diet. The best way to minimize the impact of these higher-sugar fruits is to pair them with a protein source, like prawns.

SERVES **4**

16 large raw tiger prawns, peeled
    and deveined
1 tablespoon olive oil
4 tablespoons lemon juice
2 garlic cloves, crushed
1 teaspoon grated fresh root ginger
1 teaspoon chilli powder
1 teaspoon sea salt
1 large mango, peeled, stoned and cut
    into 16 bite-sized pieces

1   Put the prawns into a large bowl and add the oil, lemon juice, garlic, ginger, chilli powder and salt. Mix well and marinate for about 10 minutes.

2   Remove the prawns from the marinade and thread 2 prawns alternately between 2 pieces of mango on each of 8 presoaked wooden skewers.

3   Place the skewers under a preheated hot grill, brush with the remaining marinade and grill for 2 minutes on each side, or until the prawns turn pink and are cooked through.

4   Serve 2 skewers per person with some dressed mixed leaf salad, if liked.

tip | Guacamole (*see page 77*) goes great alongside the skewers and provides extra fats to keep you satiated!

Red Pepper & Spring Onion Dip

Yogurt is a great staple for PCOS due to its protein content and live bacteria. If your go-to snack is a bowl of yogurt with fruit, consider mixing things up by making it savoury. This recipe completely transforms yogurt into a flavoursome dip that is perfect when paired with colourful chopped veggies.

SERVES **4**

1 large red pepper, cored, deseeded
    and quartered
2 garlic cloves, unpeeled
250 ml (8 fl oz) low-fat natural yogurt
2 spring onions, finely chopped, plus
    extra to garnish
pepper
selection of raw vegetables, such as
    carrots, cucumber, peppers, fennel,
    tomatoes, baby corn, mangetout,
    celery and courgettes, cut into batons,
    to serve

1   Slightly flatten the pepper quarters and place on a baking sheet. Wrap the garlic in foil and place on the sheet. Roast in a preheated oven, 220°C (425°F), Gas Mark 7, for 30–40 minutes until the pepper is slightly charred and the garlic is soft.

2   When cool enough to handle, remove the skin from the pepper and discard. Transfer the flesh to a bowl.

3   Squeeze the roasted garlic flesh from the cloves into the bowl.

4   Using a fork, roughly mash the pepper and garlic together. Stir in the yogurt and spring onions.

5   Garnish with extra chopped spring onion, season to taste with pepper and serve with the vegetable batons.

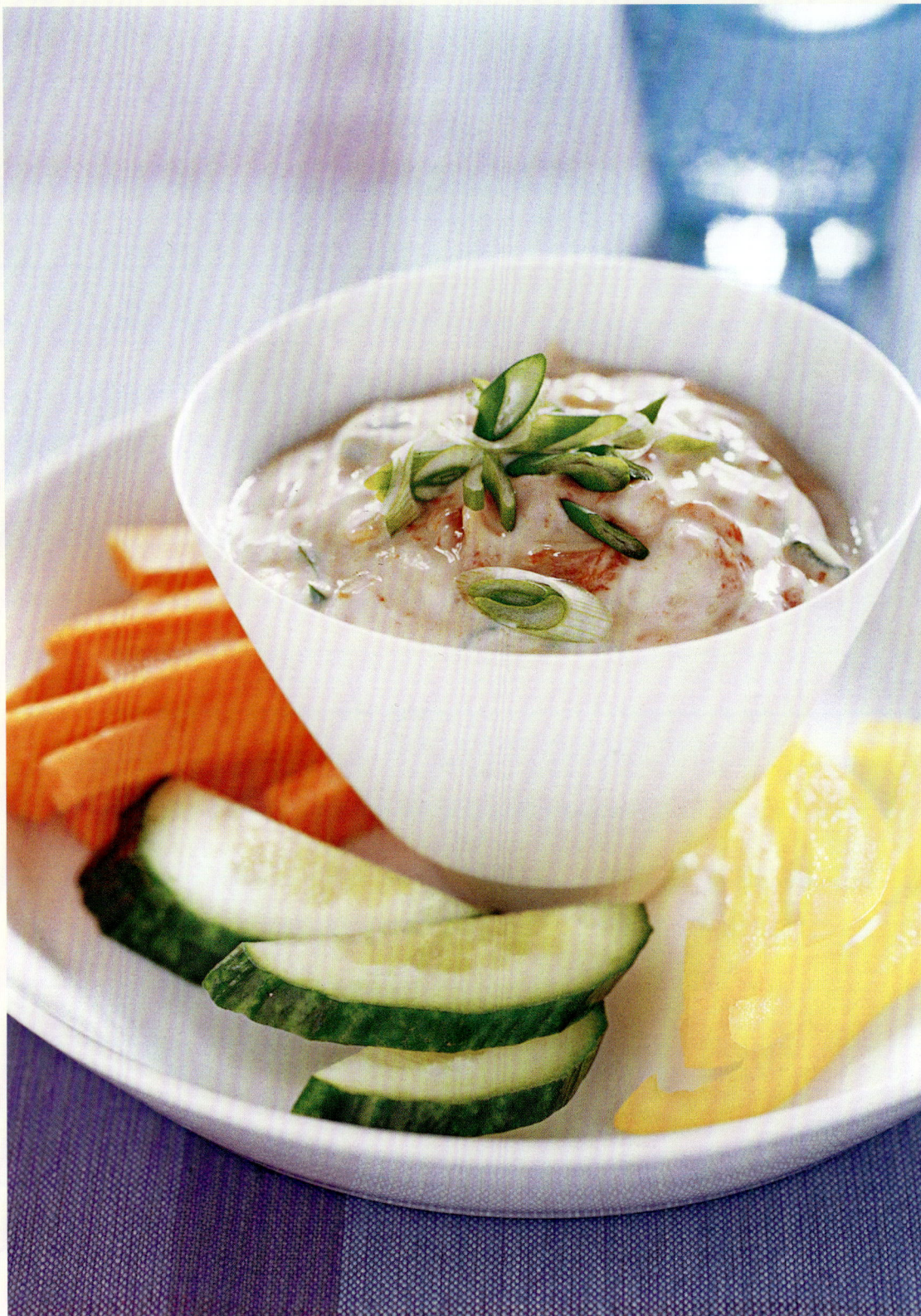

Salads
& Soups

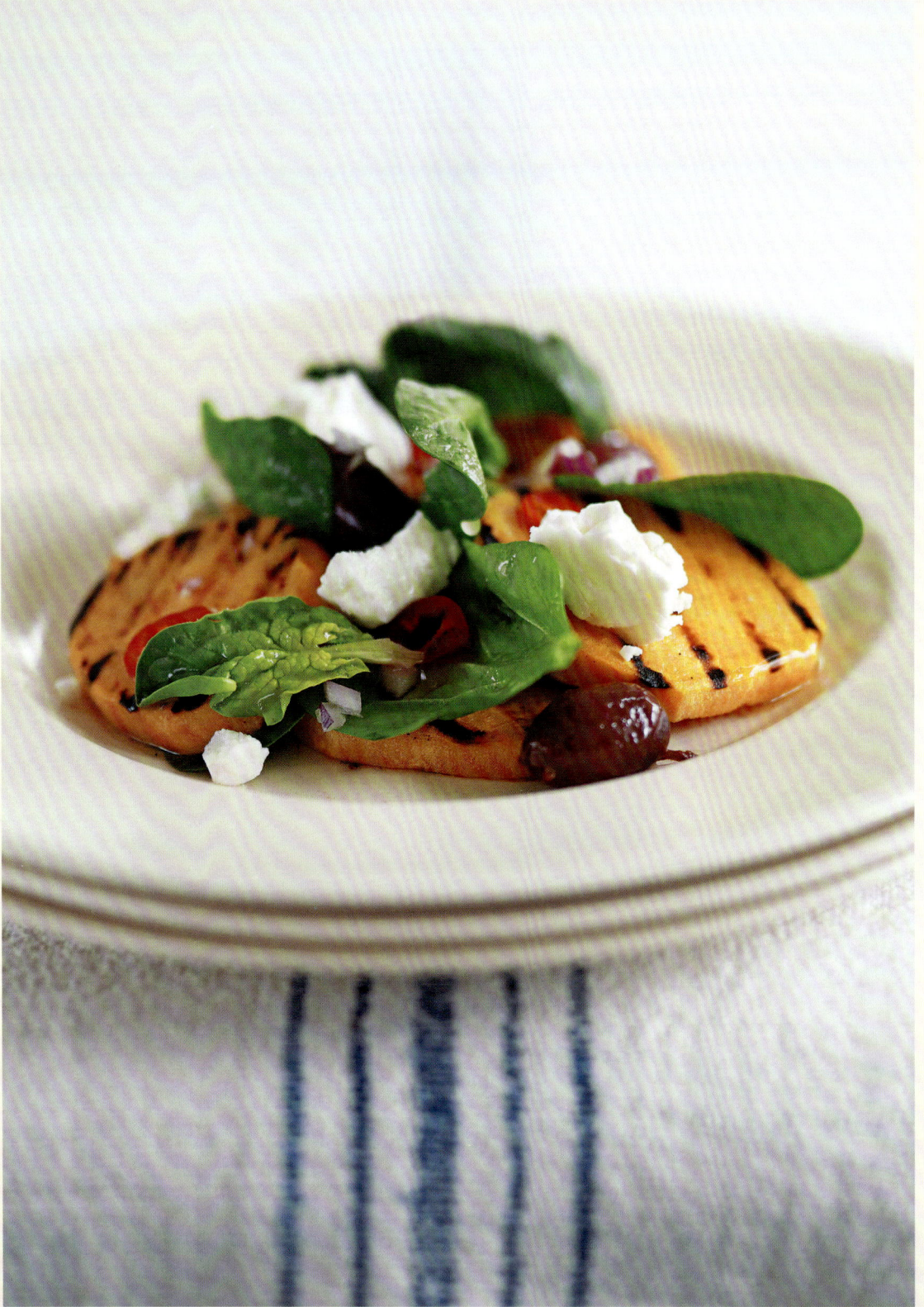

Spicy Sweet Potato & Feta Salad

Including vinegar in your meals, as a salad dressing or even taken before a carbohydrate-based dish, can help to lower the glycemic response of the meal. It's a quick hack that will help make eating to manage your PCOS a little easier!

SERVES **4**

5 tablespoons olive oil
2 sweet potatoes, thinly sliced
1 tablespoon white wine vinegar
150 g (5 oz) baby spinach leaves
1 tablespoon finely chopped red onion
125 g (4 oz) feta cheese, crumbled
1 red chilli, sliced
50 g (2 oz) pitted black olives
salt and pepper

1 Toss 2 tablespoons of the oil with the sweet potatoes. Season well and cook in a preheated hot griddle pan for 3 minutes on each side until tender and lightly charred.

2 Meanwhile, mix together the remaining oil with the white wine vinegar and season to taste. Toss with the spinach and red onion.

3 Arrange on serving plates with the sweet potatoes, feta, chilli and olives and serve immediately.

Roasted Veggie & Quinoa Salad

You can't go wrong with flavoursome, roasted vegetables. Combine with quinoa, which is high in fibre and contains some protein and a number of different B vitamins, and you have a perfect, filling lunch option. This recipe is great eaten straightaway or incorporated into meal prep.

SERVES **4**

3 courgettes, cut into chunks

2 red peppers, cored, deseeded and
    cut into chunks

2 red onions, cut into wedges

1 large aubergine, cut into chunks

3 garlic cloves, peeled

3 tablespoons olive oil

150 g (5 oz) quinoa

2 tablespoons green pesto or sun-dried
    tomato paste

1 tablespoon balsamic vinegar

75 g (3 oz) rocket leaves

1   Put all the vegetables and garlic on a large baking sheet and drizzle over the olive oil. Place in a preheated oven, 220°C (425°F), Gas Mark 7, for 20–25 minutes until tender and beginning to char.

2   Meanwhile, cook the quinoa in a saucepan of boiling water according to the packet instructions, then drain well.

3   Whisk together the pesto or tomato paste and balsamic vinegar in a small bowl. Place the roasted vegetables, rocket and quinoa in a large serving bowl and stir in the dressing. Serve warm.

tip | Add your go-to protein source to this salad, such as shredded chicken, flaked salmon, or crumbled tofu or feta.

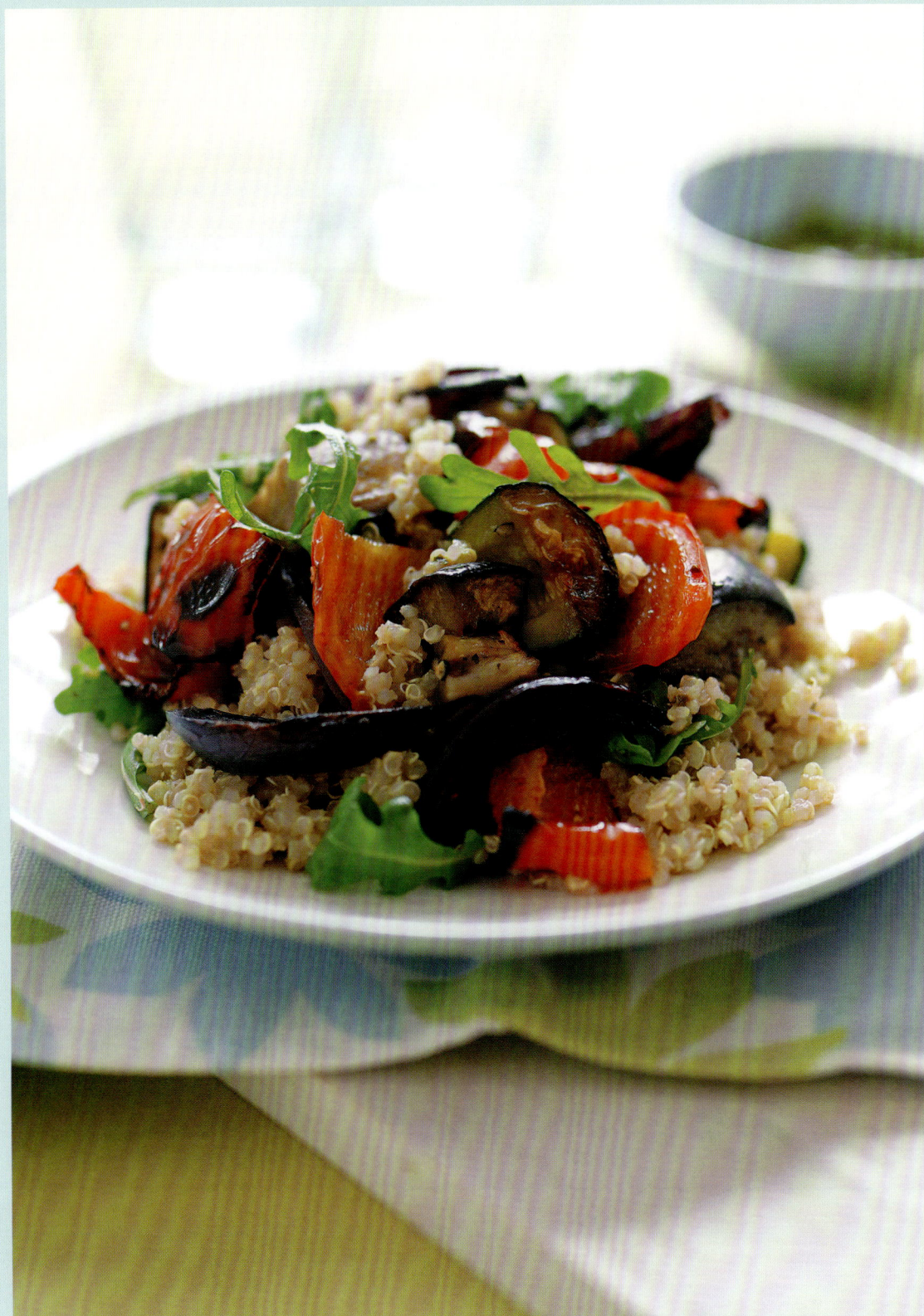

Lebanese-style Lentil & Bulgur Wheat Salad

As lentils are super-high in fibre, contain protein and have a low glycemic index, they are a great carbohydrate source to include in your PCOS-friendly meals. They also provide a number of vitamins and minerals that are supportive of PCOS, such as magnesium, folate, iron and manganese.

SERVES **4**

100 g (3½ oz) Puy lentils
1 tablespoon tomato purée
750 ml (1¼ pints) vegetable stock
100 g (3½ oz) bulgur wheat
juice of 1 lemon
1 tablespoon olive oil
2 onions, sliced
1 bunch of mint, chopped
3 tomatoes, finely chopped
salt and pepper

1   Put the lentils, tomato purée and stock in a saucepan and bring to the boil. Reduce the heat, cover tightly and simmer for 20 minutes. Add the bulgur wheat and lemon juice and season to taste with salt and pepper. Cook for 10 minutes until all the stock has been absorbed.

2   Meanwhile, heat the oil in a frying pan, add the onions and cook over a low heat until deep brown and caramelized.

3   Stir the mint into the lentil and bulgur wheat mixture, then serve warm, topped with the fried onions and chopped tomatoes.

tip | While lentils and bulgur wheat prove a good amount of plant protein, adding an extra portion of complete protein, such as feta, tofu or chicken, is a great way to keep on top of your protein intake.

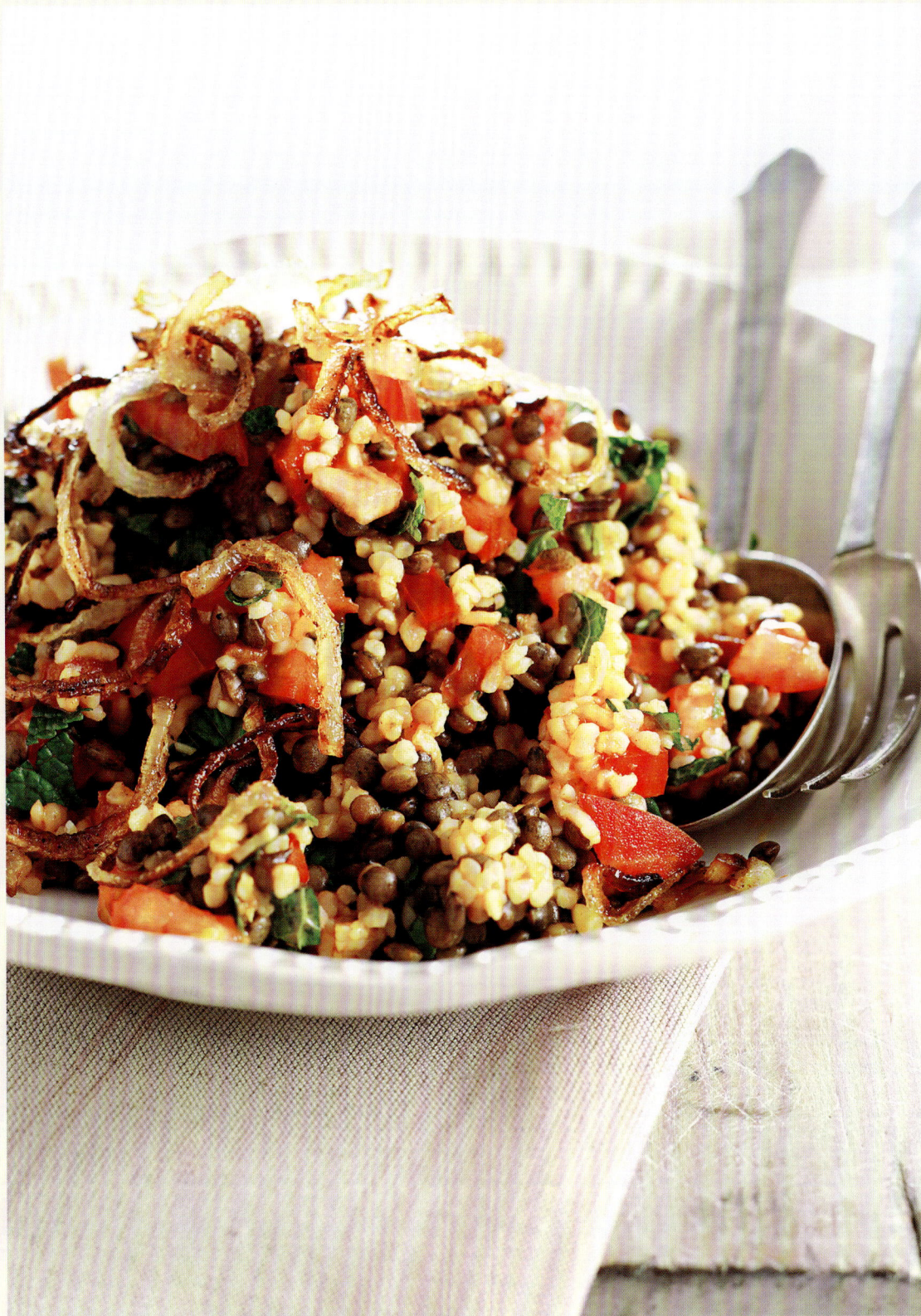

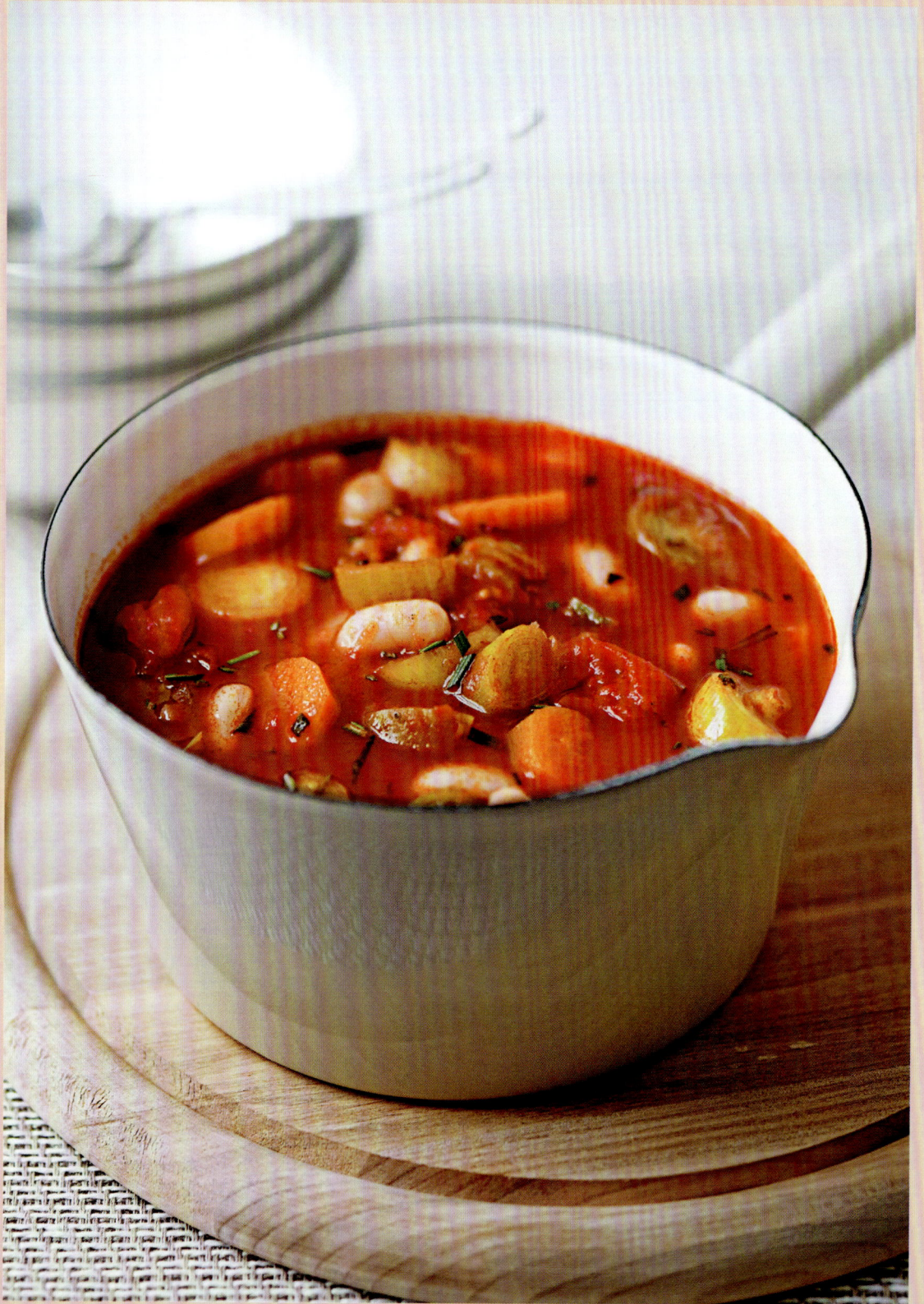

Butter Bean & Vegetable Soup

Butter beans elevate the hearty factor of any meal, especially when added to soups!
They are a great source of fibre, protein and complex carbohydrates, helping to fill you
up and support healthy cholesterol levels. They also contain folate and iron, both of which
are required for energy production.

SERVES **4**

1 tablespoon olive oil

2 teaspoons smoked paprika

1 celery stick, sliced

2 carrots, sliced

1 leek, trimmed, cleaned and sliced

600 ml (1 pint) vegetable stock

400 g (13 oz) can chopped tomatoes

400 g (13 oz) can butter beans, drained
    and rinsed

2 teaspoons chopped rosemary

salt and pepper

50 g (2 oz) vegetarian hard cheese,
    grated, to serve

1 Heat the oil in a large saucepan, add the paprika, celery, carrots and leek and cook over a medium heat for 3–4 minutes until the vegetables are slightly softened.

2 Pour over the stock and tomatoes and add the butter beans and rosemary. Season to taste with salt and pepper and bring to the boil, then cover and simmer for 15 minutes, or until the vegetables are just tender.

3 Ladle into warmed bowls and serve, sprinkled with the cheese and some freshly ground black pepper.

tip | If animal protein is a part of your diet, add some shredded chicken to boost this dish's nutritional density.

Lentil & Feta Salad

Puy lentils are a great way to turn up the heartiness factor of any vegetarian meal. They are meaty and dense, and a great source of plant protein to keep you satiated. Puy lentils contain good amounts of polyphenols, a plant compound with antioxidant properties that may help to reduce the risk of cardiovascular disease. They also contain folate, which contributes to a healthy nervous system and energy production.

SERVES **2–4**

250 g (8 oz) Puy lentils
2 carrots, finely diced
2 celery sticks, finely diced
100 g (3½ oz) feta cheese
2 tablespoons chopped parsley
salt and pepper

DRESSING

3 tablespoons white wine vinegar
2 teaspoons Dijon mustard
5 tablespoons olive oil

1   Put the lentils in a saucepan, cover with cold water and add a pinch of salt. Bring to the boil and cook for 20–25 minutes until just cooked but not mushy. Drain and refresh in cold water, then drain again and transfer to a large salad bowl.

2   Add the carrots and celery to the bowl with the lentils. Crumble in the feta and add the chopped parsley.

3   Make the dressing by whisking together the vinegar, mustard and oil.

4   Add the dressing to the salad and stir to combine well. Season to taste with salt and pepper and serve immediately.

tip | No feta to hand? Crumbled tofu would work well here too.

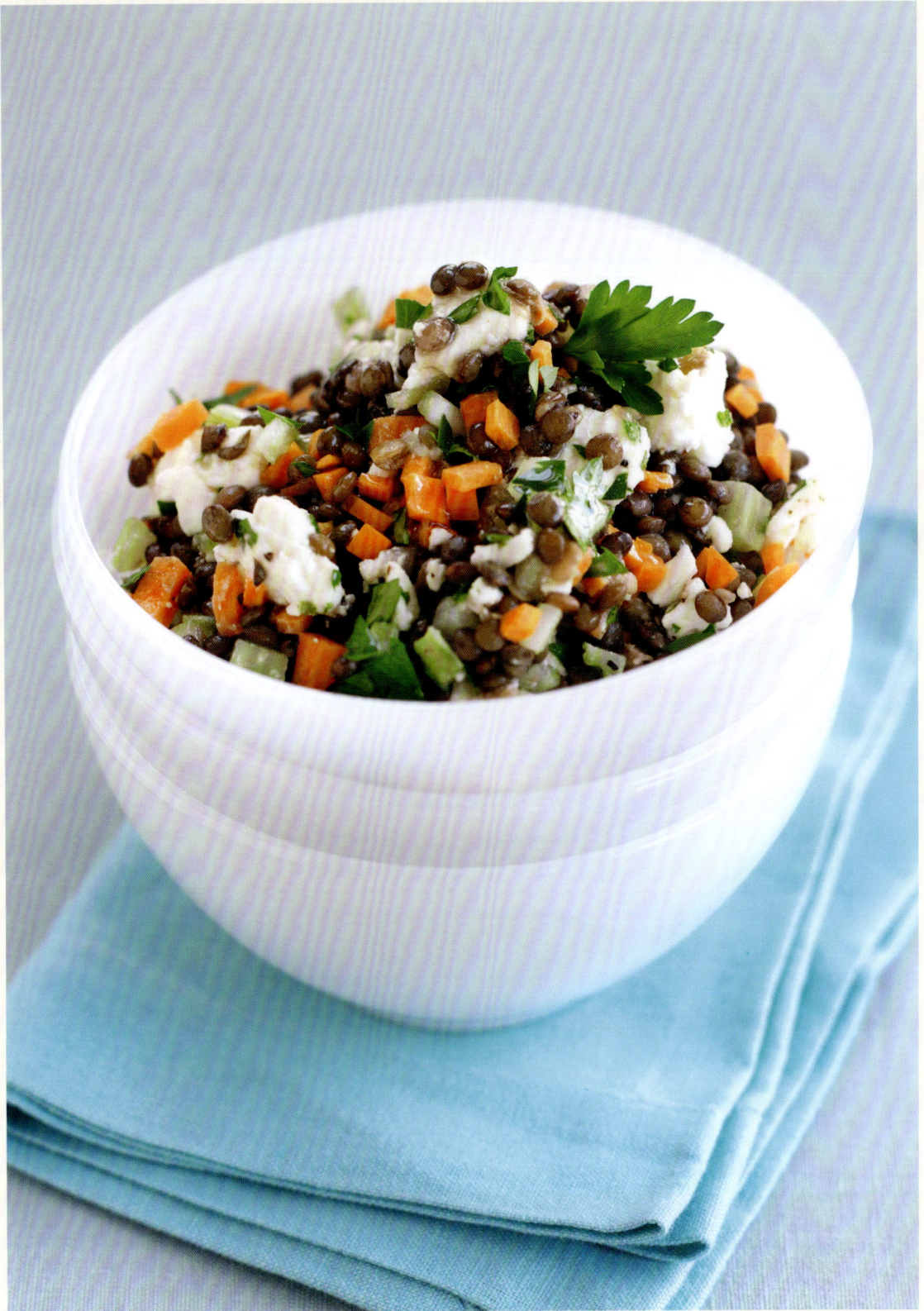

Carrot, Lentil & Tahini Soup

Soups are a great way to pack in a number of different nutrient-dense plants, protein and healthy fats, and they can be meal-prepped ahead of the week. Adding tahini or Greek yogurt to a veggie-packed soup is a great way to add a little creaminess and extra healthy fats to keep you full and satisfied.

SERVES 4

2 tablespoons sesame seeds, plus extra
    for sprinkling
2 tablespoons olive oil
1 onion, chopped
500 g (1 lb) carrots, chopped
1 litre (1¾ pints) vegetable stock
2 teaspoons chopped lemon thyme
    leaves, plus extra for sprinkling
150 g (5 oz) dried green lentils, rinsed
    and drained
5 tablespoons tahini paste
Greek yogurt, for topping
salt and pepper

1   Heat the sesame seeds in a large dry saucepan until lightly toasted. Tip out into a small bowl.

2   Add the oil to the pan and gently fry the onion and carrots for 10 minutes until softened. Add the stock and thyme and bring to the boil. Reduce the heat, cover and cook very gently for 10 minutes.

3   Tip in the lentils, cover and cook gently for a further 20 minutes, or until the lentils are soft.

4   Remove from the heat and leave to stand for 5 minutes, then stir in the tahini paste. Season to taste with salt and pepper.

5   Ladle into bowls and top with spoonfuls of Greek yogurt. Serve sprinkled with extra sesame seeds and thyme leaves.

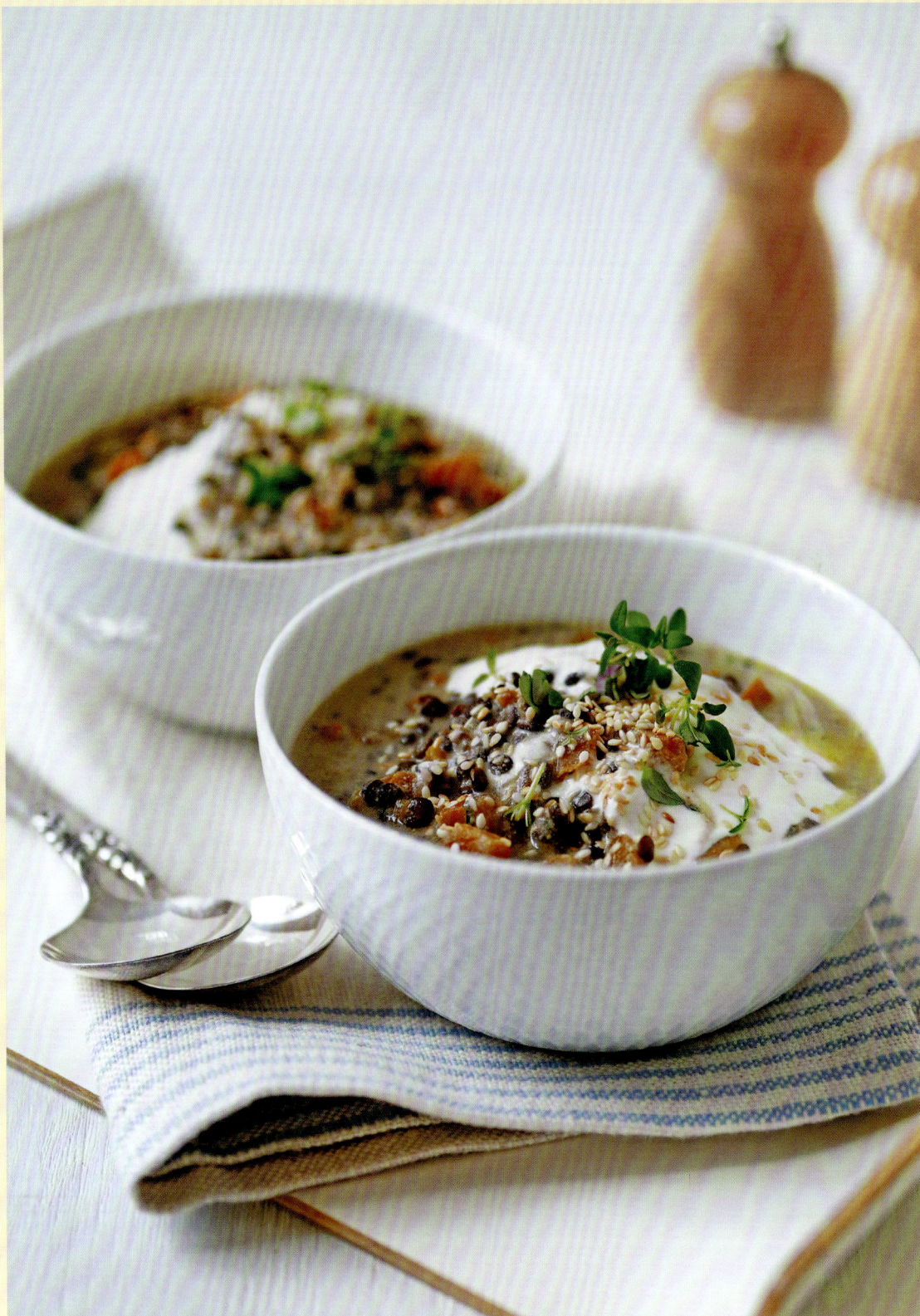

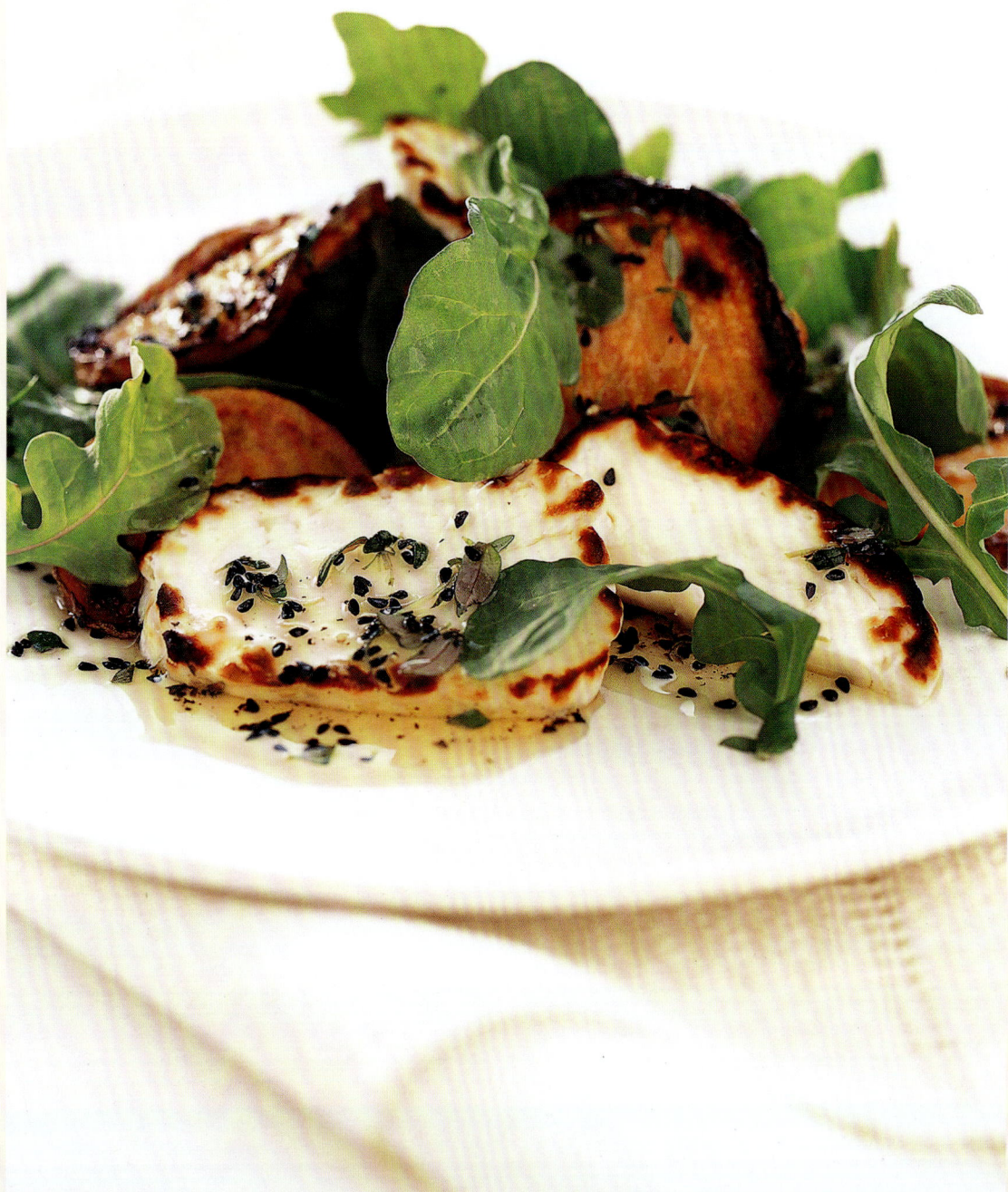

Sweet Potato & Halloumi Salad

Due to their high fibre content, sweet potatoes are considered a complex carbohydrate, digested and broken down into glucose more slowly than refined carbs, which helps to control the body's insulin response. Add a source of protein like halloumi and some healthy fats for the perfect PCOS meal formula.

SERVES 4

500 g (1 lb) sweet potatoes, sliced
3 tablespoons olive oil, plus extra
    for greasing
250 g (8 oz) halloumi cheese, thinly sliced
75 g (3 oz) rocket leaves

DRESSING

5 tablespoons olive oil
2 tablespoons runny honey
2 tablespoons lemon or lime juice
1½ teaspoons black onion seeds
1 red chilli, deseeded and finely sliced
2 teaspoons chopped lemon thyme
salt and pepper

1   Mix together all the ingredients for the dressing in a small bowl. Set aside until required.

2   Cook the sweet potatoes in a saucepan of lightly salted boiling water for 2 minutes. Drain well and chill until required.

3   When ready to serve, heat the oil in a large frying pan, add the sweet potatoes and fry for about 10 minutes, turning once, until golden.

4   Meanwhile, place the halloumi slices on a lightly oiled foil-lined grill rack. Cook under a preheated medium grill for about 3 minutes until golden.

5   Divide the sweet potatoes, cheese and rocket among 4 serving plates and spoon over the dressing. Serve immediately.

Mackerel & Wild Rice Niçoise

Swapping regular white rice for wild rice is a super-simple way to boost the both the fibre and antioxidant profile of a meal. While it may take a little longer to cook, the health benefits you'll gain are definitely worth it. Pair with colourful vegetables, dark leafy green vegetables and an omega-3-rich oily fish, such as mackerel, as your protein source and you have a great PCOS-friendly meal.

SERVES **3–4**

100 g (3½ oz) wild rice

150 g (5 oz) green beans, halved

300 g (10 oz) large mackerel fillets, pin-boned

6 tablespoons olive oil

12 black olives

8 canned anchovy fillets, drained and halved

250 g (8 oz) cherry tomatoes, halved

3 hard-boiled eggs, cut into quarters

1 tablespoon lemon juice

1 tablespoon French mustard

2 tablespoons chopped chives

salt and pepper

1 Cook the rice in plenty of boiling water for 20–25 minutes, or until it is tender. (The grains will start to split open when they're just cooked.) Add the green beans and cook for 2 minutes.

2 Meanwhile, lay the mackerel on a foil-lined grill rack and brush with 1 tablespoon of the oil. Cook under a preheated hot grill for 8–10 minutes, or until cooked through. Leave to cool.

3 Drain the rice and beans and mix together in a salad bowl with the olives, anchovies, tomatoes and eggs. Flake the mackerel, discarding any stray bones, and add to the bowl.

4 Mix the remaining oil with the lemon juice, mustard, chives and a little salt and pepper, and add to the bowl. Toss the ingredients lightly together, cover and chill until ready to serve.

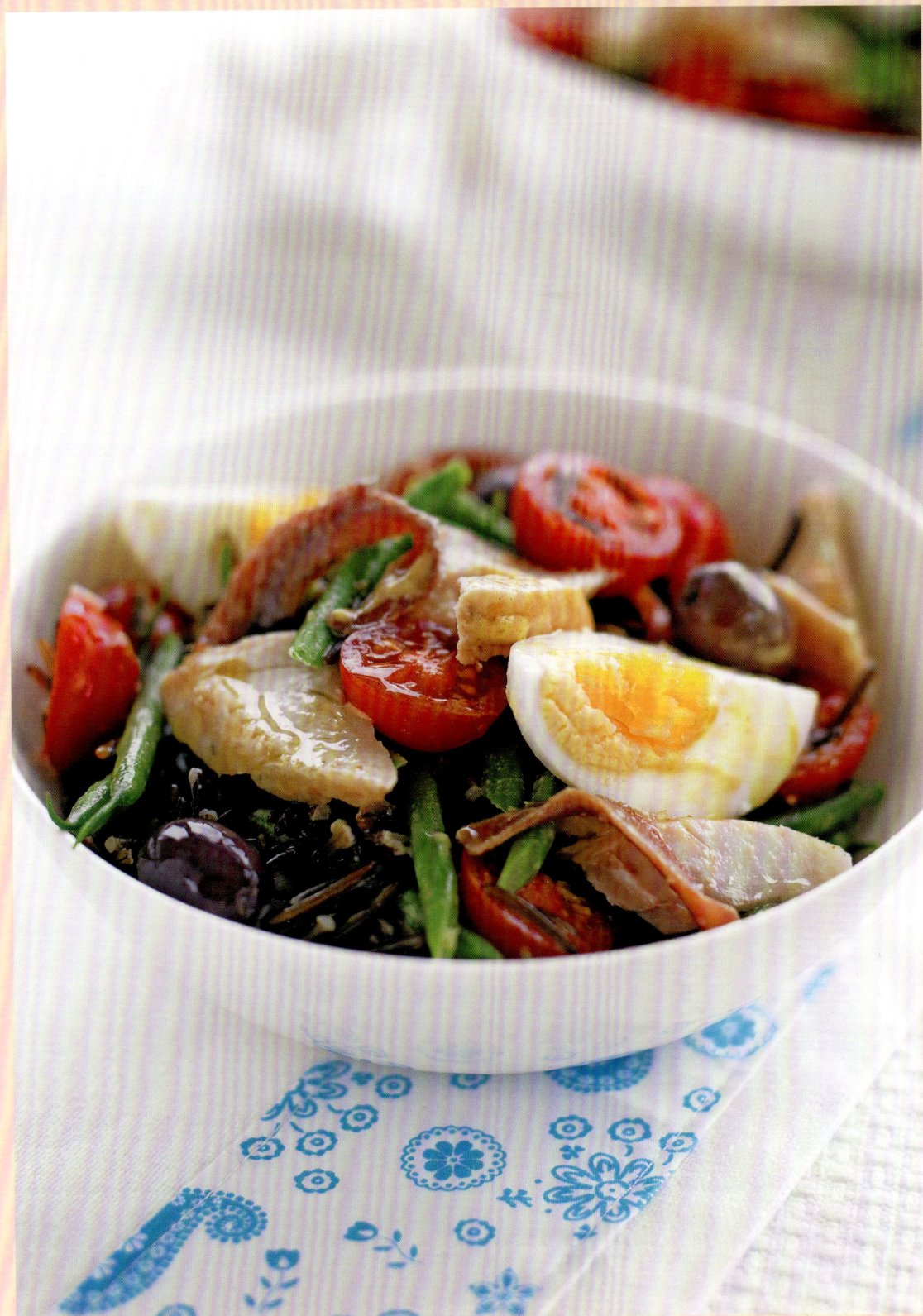

Salmon & Chickpea Salad

This salad is nutritious, fresh and packed full of flavour. It will make a great addition to your salad repertoire. Chickpeas contain B6, a member of the vitamin B family, which helps the regulation of hormonal activity. It also helps us to produce the neurotransmitter GABA, which is calming, and serotonin, which impacts mood.

SERVES 4

625 g (1¼ lb) salmon fillet, skinned
1 orange
grated zest of ½ lemon
2 tablespoons extra virgin olive oil
400 g (13 oz) can chickpeas, rinsed
    and drained
60 g (2¼ oz) watercress
2 tablespoons caper berries, rinsed
    and drained
small handful of mint leaves, roughly torn
salt and pepper

1 Cook the salmon under a preheated hot grill for 8–9 minutes, turning once, or until cooked through.

2 Meanwhile, grate the zest of the orange into a bowl, then peel and segment the orange, catching the juice in the bowl. Whisk together the orange juice and zest, grated lemon zest, oil and some salt and pepper.

3 Flake the salmon in large pieces into a serving bowl. Toss together with the remaining ingredients and the orange segments and dressing, then serve.

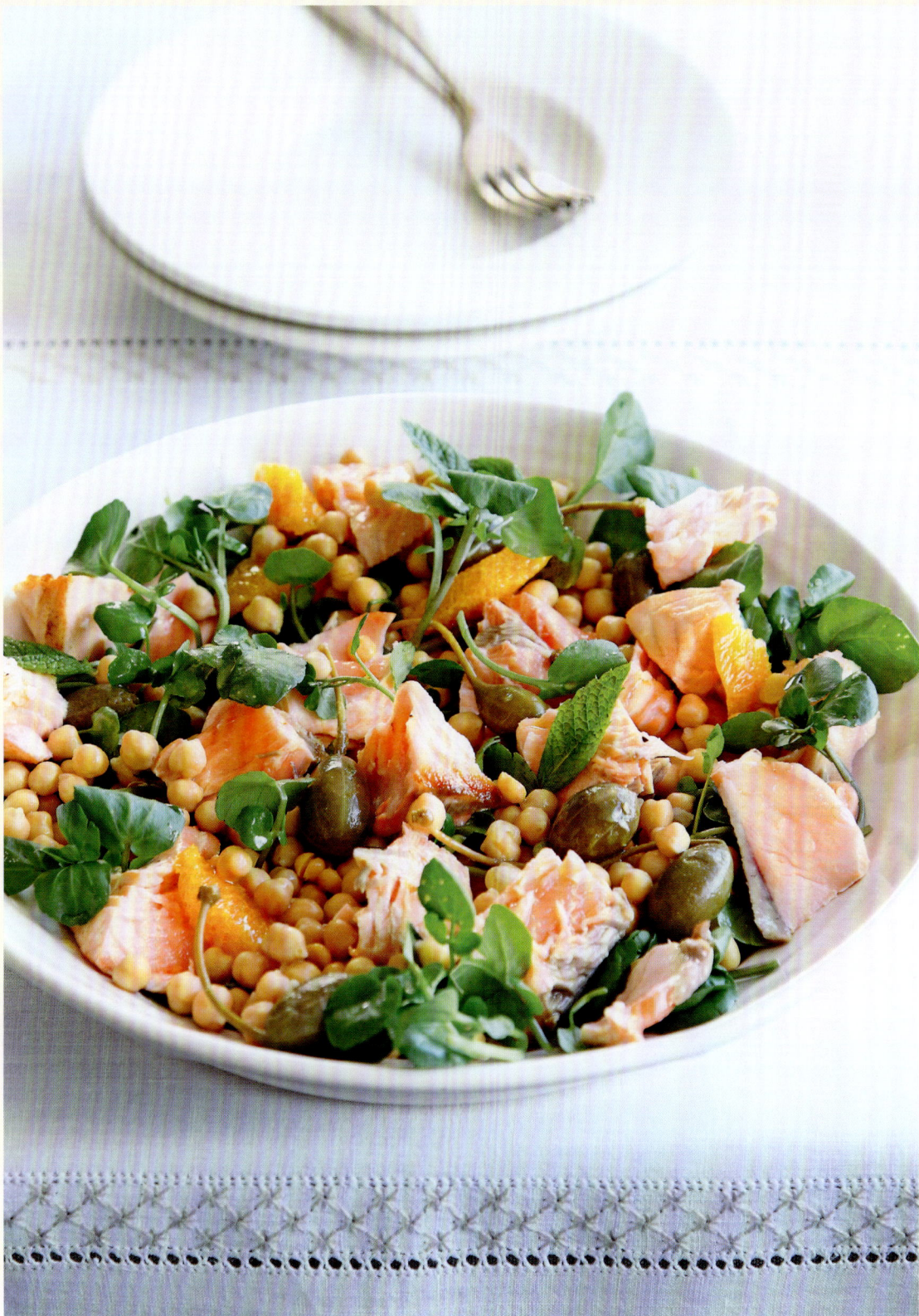

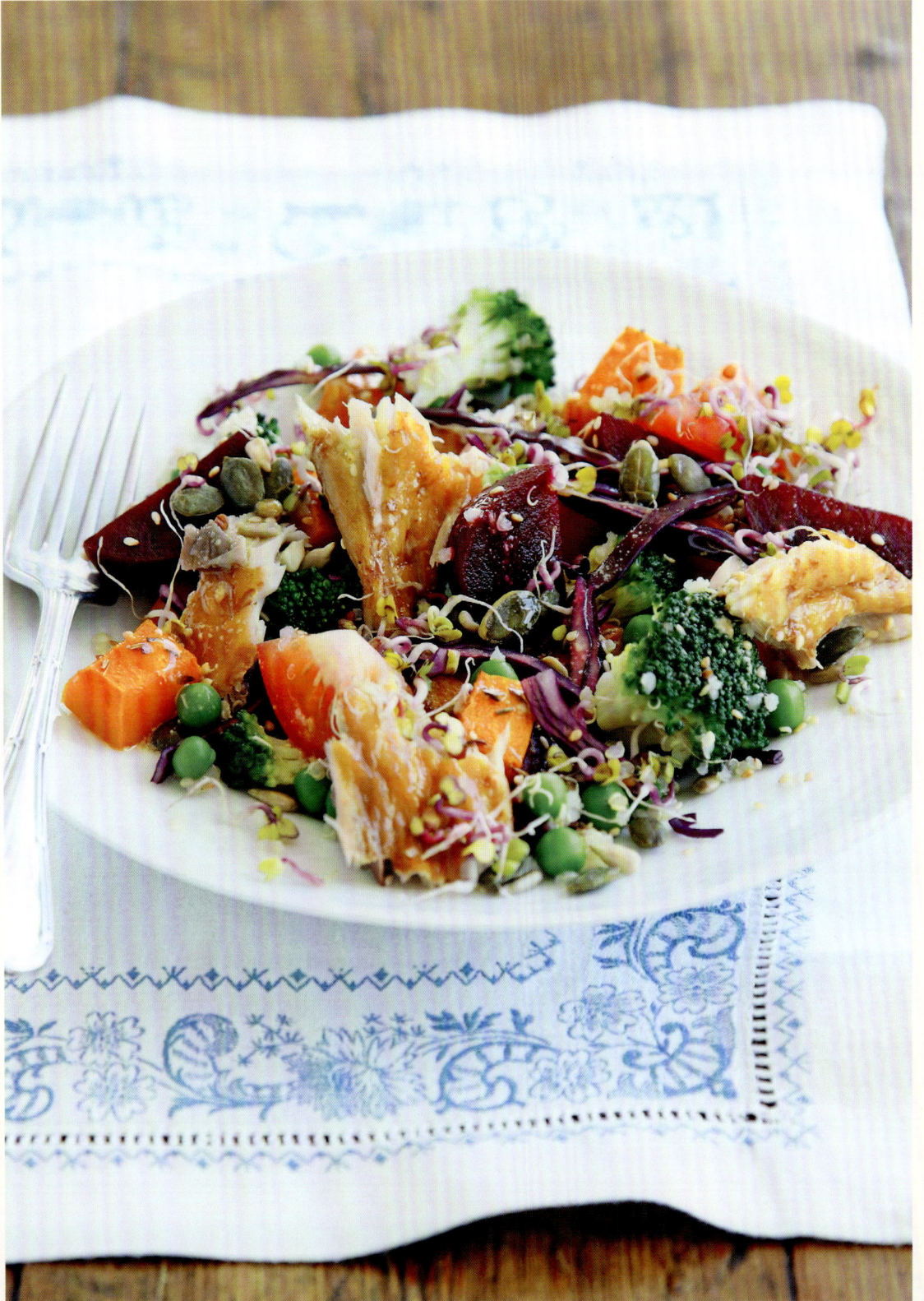

Smoked Mackerel Superfood Salad

Mackerel is rich in anti-inflammatory omega-3 fatty acids, specifically Eicosapentaenoic acid (EPA) and Docosahexaenoic acid (DHA). DHA plays an important role in maintaining brain health and can support mental wellbeing by reducing symptoms of depression and anxiety. Add to a colourful, high-fibre super salad and you have the perfect PCOS lunch.

SERVES **2**

500 g (1 lb) butternut squash, peeled, deseeded and cut into 1-cm (½-inch) cubes

4 tablespoons olive oil

1 teaspoon cumin seeds

1 head of broccoli, cut into florets

200 g (7 oz) frozen or fresh peas

3 tablespoons quinoa

4 tablespoons mixed seeds

2 smoked mackerel fillets

juice of 1 lemon

½ teaspoon honey

½ teaspoon Dijon mustard

100 g (3½ oz) red cabbage, shredded

4 tomatoes, chopped

4 cooked beetroot, cut into wedges

20 g (¾ oz) radish sprouts

1 Place the squash in a roasting tin. Sprinkle with 1 tablespoon of the oil and the cumin seeds. Cook in a preheated oven, 200°C (400°F), Gas Mark 6, for 15–18 minutes until tender. Set aside.

2 Meanwhile, cook the broccoli in boiling water for 4–5 minutes until tender, adding the peas 3 minutes before the end of the cooking time. Remove with a slotted spoon and refresh under cold running water, then drain. Cook the quinoa in the broccoli water for 15 minutes. Drain and let cool slightly.

3 Heat a nonstick frying pan over a medium-low heat and dry-fry the seeds, stirring frequently, until golden brown and toasted. Set aside. Heat the mackerel fillets according to the pack instructions, then skin and break into flakes.

4 Whisk together the remaining olive oil, lemon juice, honey and mustard in a small bowl.

5 Toss all the ingredients, except the sprouts, with the dressing in a serving bowl. Top with the sprouts to serve.

Seared Salmon
with Avocado Salad

Increasing your intake of omega-3 fatty acids can do wonders for PCOS symptoms, and this salmon and avocado salad is a tasty way to do just that. Oily fish, including salmon, contains high amounts of omega-3, which has been shown to improve insulin resistance and triglyceride levels and aid mental wellness. Supplementing omega-3 has also been shown to improve fertility in those with PCOS.

SERVES 4

2 tablespoons olive oil

4 pieces of salmon fillet, about 200 g
   (7 oz) each, skin on and pin-boned

1 large orange

2 tablespoons extra virgin olive oil

salt and pepper

AVOCADO SALAD

2 ripe avocados, peeled and cut into
   1-cm (½-inch) dice

1 red chilli, deseeded and finely chopped

juice of 1 lime

1 tablespoon roughly chopped coriander

1 tablespoon olive oil

1   Heat a small frying pan over a high heat. When the pan is hot, add the olive oil. Season the salmon fillets with salt and pepper and place them, skin-side down, in the pan. Cook for 4 minutes, then turn the fish over and cook for a further 2 minutes.

2   Heat another small frying pan on the hob. Zest the orange into strips and set aside, then cut it in half and place the orange halves, cut-sides down, in the pan. Sear until they start to blacken. Remove the oranges from the pan, then squeeze their juice into the pan. Bring the juice to the boil and reduce it until you have around 1 tablespoon left. Whisk in the extra virgin olive oil and season with salt and pepper.

3   For the salad, place the avocados in a mixing bowl, add the remaining ingredients and season to taste.

4   To serve, spoon the avocado salad onto each plate alongside a piece of salmon, drizzle with the orange vinaigrette and sprinkle with a little of the orange zest.

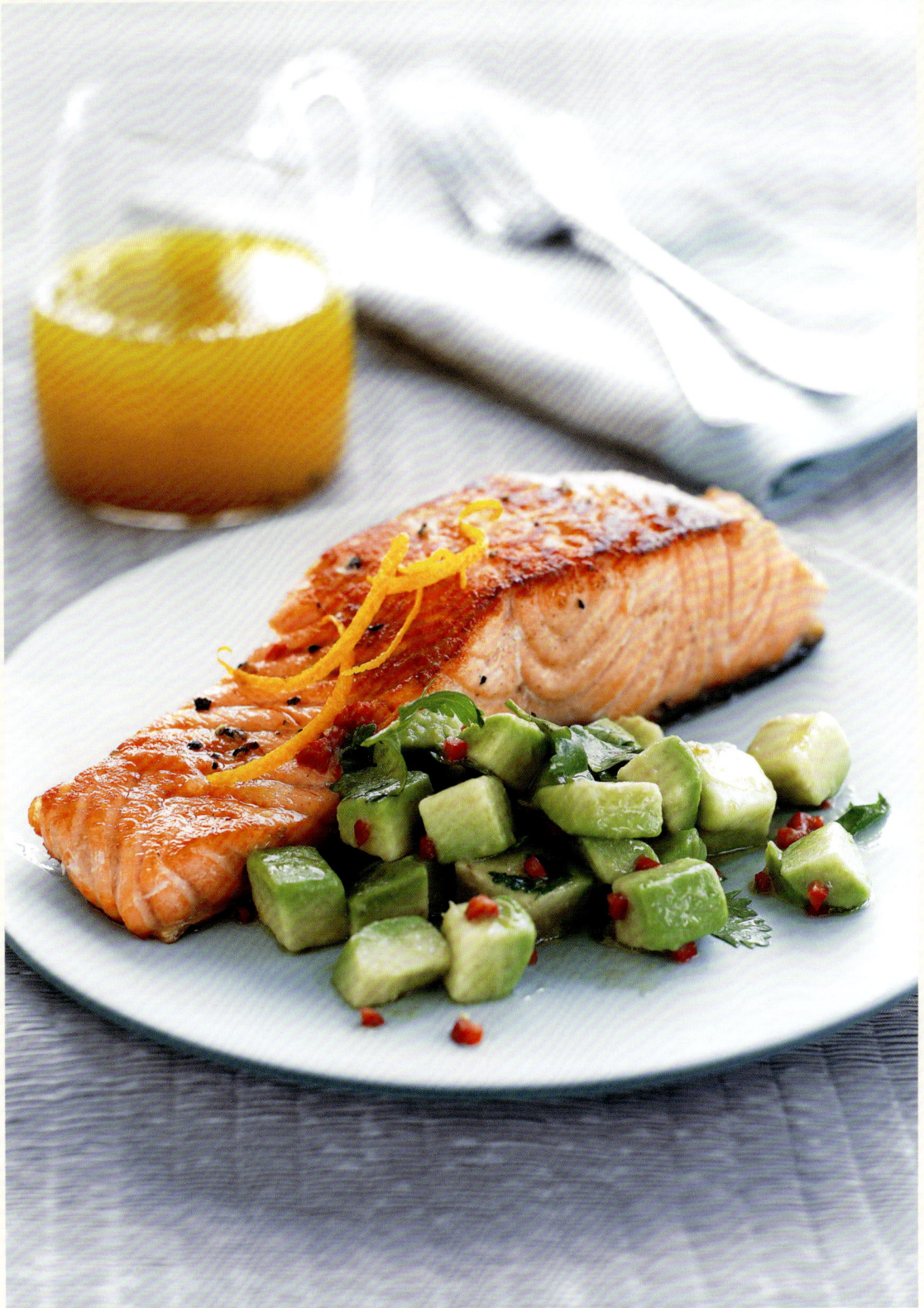

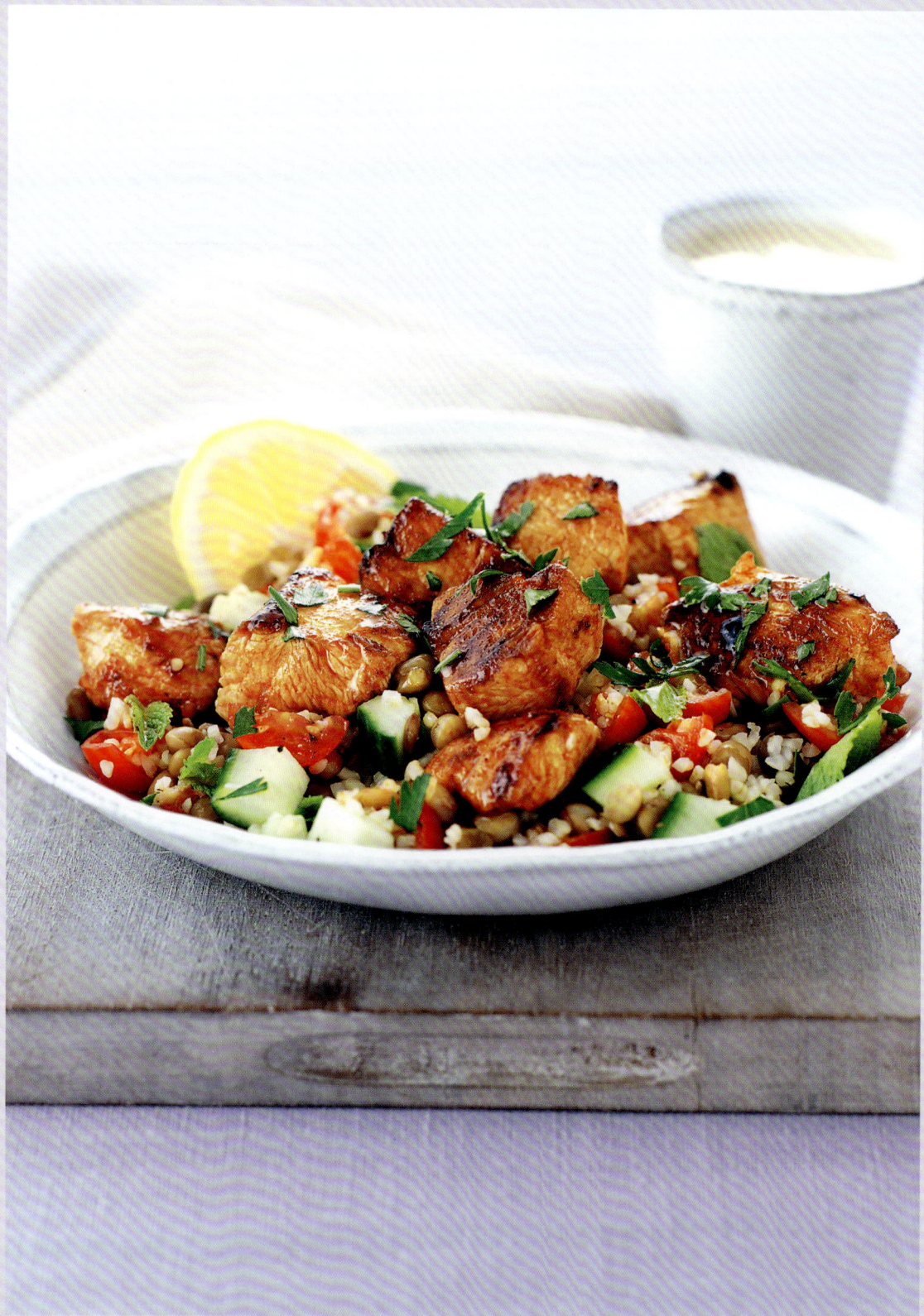

Turkey Skewers
with Bulgur Wheat Salad

Turkey is a fantastic protein source to base your PCOS-healthy meals around. It is rich in the amino acid tryptophan, which gets converted into both melatonin, our sleep hormone, and serotonin, a neurotransmitter that influences our mood.

SERVES **4**

2 tablespoons olive oil

2 tablespoons lemon juice

1 teaspoon paprika

3 tablespoons chopped flat leaf parsley, plus extra to garnish

400 g (13 oz) turkey breast, diced

salt and pepper

BULGUR WHEAT SALAD

400 ml (14 fl oz) chicken stock

250 g (8 oz) bulgur wheat

410 g (13½ oz) can green lentils, rinsed and drained

½ cucumber

10 cherry tomatoes

20 g (¾ oz) mint, chopped

lemon wedges, to garnish

HUMMUS DRESSING

4 tablespoons hummus

1 tablespoon lemon juice

1 tablespoon water

1 Presoak 8 wooden skewers in warm water. Mix together the oil, lemon juice, paprika and parsley, and season to taste. Add the turkey and turn in the mixture to coat thoroughly. Set aside for at least 20 minutes.

2 Drain the turkey (discard any marinade) and thread the pieces on to the skewers. Cook under a preheated hot grill, turning once or twice, for 10 minutes, or until cooked through.

3 Meanwhile, bring the stock to the boil and cook the bulgur wheat according to the instructions on the packet. Drain and spread out to cool. Stir in the green lentils, cucumber, tomatoes and mint.

4 Make the dressing by combining the hummus with the lemon juice and water.

5 Serve the turkey skewers with the bulgur wheat salad, garnished with lemon wedges and flat leaf parsley. Offer the dressing separately.

tip | Gluten-free? Swap the bulgur wheat for quinoa, buckwheat or brown rice.

Wild Rice & Turkey Salad

Adding fruit to a salad alongside a source of protein and fat, like this wild rice and turkey salad, helps to slow the release of the natural sugars from the fruit, and keep your blood glucose levels stable. Added fruit like apple also brings a different flavour and texture to your salads, keeping things interesting at lunchtime.

SERVES **4**

300 g (10 oz) wild rice
2 green apples, finely sliced
75 g (3 oz) pecan nuts
rind and juice of 2 oranges
60 g (2¼ oz) cranberries
3 tablespoons olive oil
2 tablespoons chopped parsley
4 turkey fillets, each about 125 g (4 oz)
salt and pepper

1   Cook the rice according to the instructions on the packet and allow to cool to room temperature.

2   Mix the apples into the rice with the pecans, the orange rind and juice and the cranberries. Season to taste with salt and pepper.

3   Mix together the oil and parsley. Cut the turkey fillets into halves or thirds lengthways and cover with this mixture. Heat a frying pan until it is hot but not smoking and cook the turkey fillets for 2 minutes on each side. Slice the turkey, arrange the pieces next to the rice salad and serve immediately.

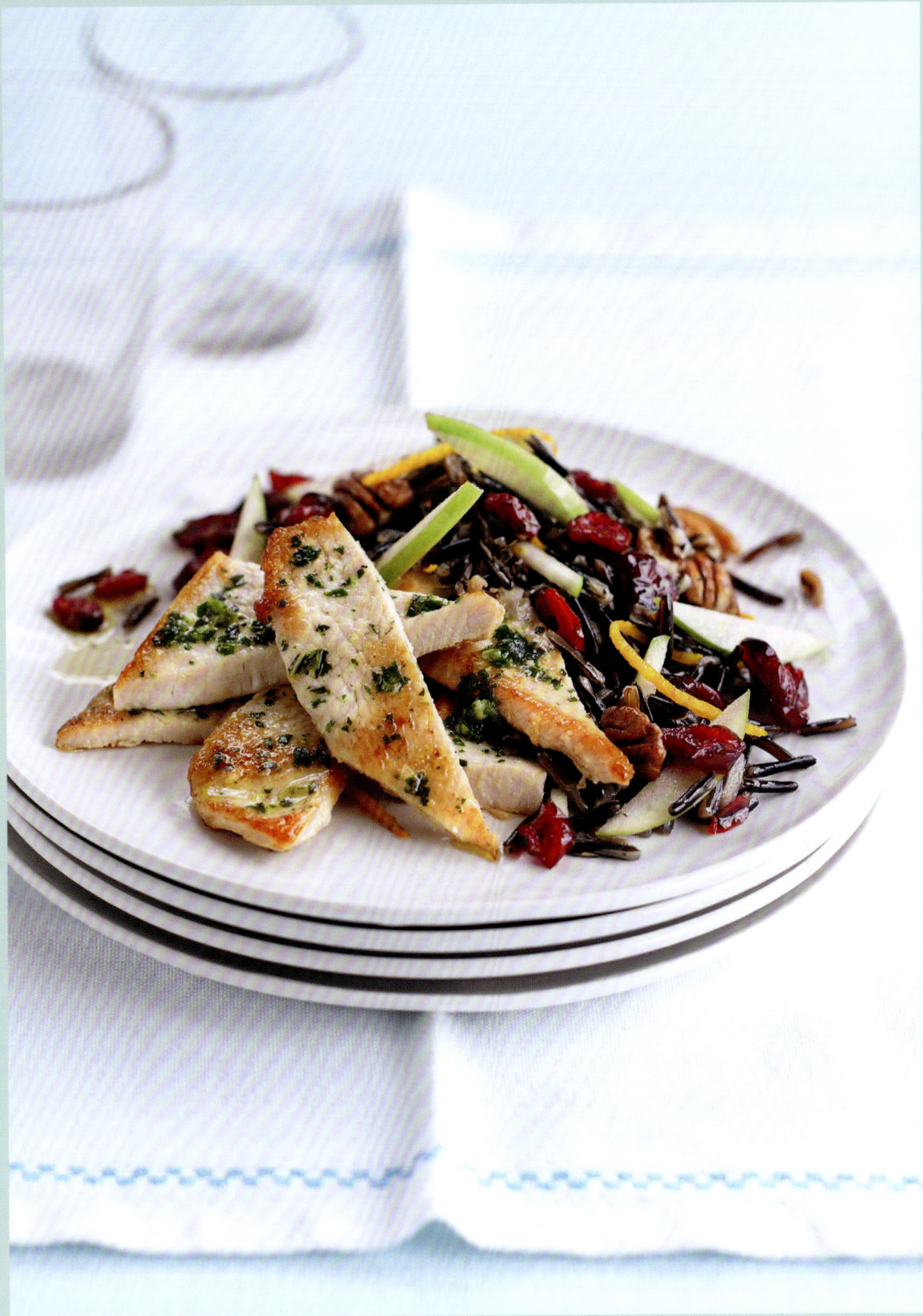

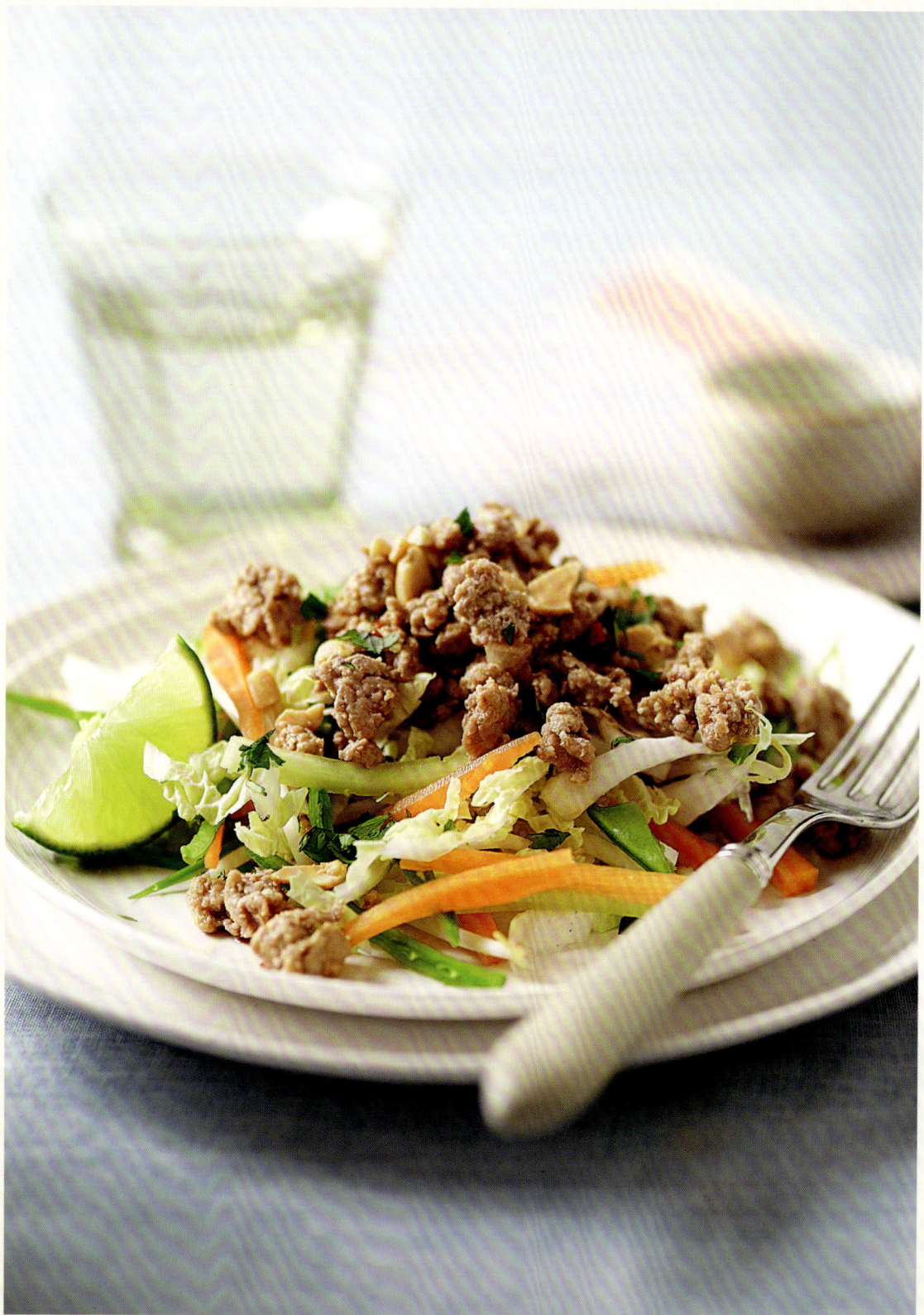

Minced Turkey Salad
with Lime & Ginger Dressing

A low-carb diet has been shown to be beneficial for those with PCOS, helping to improve a number of symptoms and reduce certain risk factors. Having delicious low-carb, high-fibre recipes in your repertoire can help make managing your PCOS feel less overwhelming, and this turkey salad is a great example of that.

SERVES **4**

500 g (1 lb) minced turkey

2 garlic cloves, finely chopped

1 shallot, finely chopped

1 small red chilli, deseeded and
   finely chopped

1½ tablespoons olive oil

½ Chinese cabbage, shredded

150 g (5 oz) mangetout, shredded

½ small cucumber, cut into thin
   matchsticks

250 g (8 oz) bean sprouts

1 carrot, peeled and cut into thin
   matchsticks

3 spring onions, thinly sliced

4 tablespoons unsalted peanuts, chopped

chopped coriander, to garnish

lime wedges, to serve

LIME & GINGER DRESSING

1½ teaspoons peeled and grated fresh
   root ginger

1½ teaspoons fish sauce

1 tablespoon light soy sauce

2 tablespoons lime juice

2 tablespoons sesame oil

1   Mix together the turkey, garlic, shallot and chilli in a bowl. Heat the olive oil in a large frying pan over a medium-high heat, add the turkey mixture and stir-fry for 8–10 minutes, or until the meat is browned and cooked through. Tip into a large bowl.

2   Whisk together all of the dressing ingredients in a small bowl and pour over the cooked turkey. Leave to cool for 10 minutes.

3   Meanwhile, mix together the Chinese cabbage, mangetout, cucumber, bean sprouts, carrot and spring onions in a bowl. Pile on to serving plates and spoon over the turkey. Sprinkle with the peanuts and coriander and serve immediately with lime wedges on the side.

Quinoa Salad
with Seared Chicken

Wholegrains are a staple of a healthy PCOS diet. They are a complex carbohydrate source, which means that they help to keep blood sugar levels more stable compared to refined carbohydrates. Wholegrains like quinoa also contain a variety of different micronutrients, such as magnesium, which aids insulin sensitivity and reduces blood pressure, and zinc, which can help lower androgen activity, therefore reducing PCOS symptoms.

SERVES **4**

175 g (6 oz) quinoa
¼ cucumber, finely diced
1 small green pepper, cored, deseeded
    and finely diced
6 spring onions, trimmed, thinly sliced
125 g (4 oz) frozen peas, just defrosted
grated zest and juice of 1 lemon
2 tablespoons olive oil
1 tablespoon harissa paste
4 boneless, skinless chicken breasts,
    cut into long thin slices
small bunch mint, finely chopped

DRESSING

3 tablespoons olive oil
1 tablespoon harissa paste
grated zest and juice of 1 lemon
salt

1   Add the quinoa to a saucepan of boiling water and simmer for about 10 minutes, or according to the packet instructions, until just tender, then drain in a fine sieve.

2   Make the dressing by mixing the olive oil, harissa, lemon zest and juice and a little salt in a salad bowl. Stir in the hot quinoa and leave to cool, then mix in the cucumber, green pepper, spring onions and frozen peas.

3   Mix the lemon zest and juice, oil and harissa in a shallow bowl, then add the chicken and toss well. Heat a griddle pan (or ordinary frying pan) over a medium heat and cook the chicken in batches for about 6 minutes, turning until browned on both sides and cooked through.

4   Stir the mint through the quinoa salad, then top with the warm chicken. Serve warm or cold. Any leftovers can be chilled and packed into lunchboxes the following day.

SALADS & SOUPS

116

Beef & Barley Broth

On cold evenings, nothing beats a hearty beef stew. Beef's high iron content is great for supporting energy levels, but it also contains a number of other key minerals and vitamins that help us thrive every day with PCOS, such as folate, copper, zinc and vitamin A.

SERVES **6**

25 g (1 oz) butter

250 g (8 oz) braising beef, fat trimmed away and meat cut into small cubes

1 large onion, finely chopped

200 g (7 oz) swede, diced

150 g (5 oz) carrot, diced

100 g (3½ oz) pearl barley

2 litres (3½ pints) beef bone broth

2 teaspoons dry English mustard (optional)

salt and pepper

chopped parsley, to garnish

1   Heat the butter in a large saucepan, add the beef and onion and fry for 5 minutes, stirring, until the beef is browned and the onion just beginning to colour.

2   Stir in the diced vegetables, pearl barley, stock and mustard, if using. Season with salt and pepper and bring to the boil. Cover and simmer for 1¾ hours, stirring occasionally until the meat and vegetables are very tender.

3   Taste and adjust the seasoning, if needed. Ladle the soup into bowls and sprinkle with a little chopped parsley. Serve with sourdough bread.

Light
Lunches

Curried Tofu
with Vegetables

If you opt for a plant-based diet and are conscious of your protein intake, tofu is a great staple to have in your kitchen. Unlike legumes, it is a complete protein source and low in carbohydrates, helping to keep blood sugar levels stable while also supporting healthy muscle function.

SERVES **4**

2 tablespoons olive oil

2 teaspoons finely grated fresh root ginger

8 garlic cloves, chopped

8 small shallots, chopped

1 teaspoon ground turmeric

2 red chillies, chopped

4 tablespoons very finely chopped
    lemon grass

400 ml (14 fl oz) coconut milk

200 ml (7 fl oz) vegetable stock

4 lime leaves, finely shredded

12 baby courgettes, cut in half lengthways

12 baby sweetcorn, trimmed and cut
    in half lengthways

400 g (13 oz) firm tofu, cut into
    bite-sized cubes

1 tablespoon dark soy sauce

1 tablespoon lime juice

small handful of finely chopped
    fresh coriander

salt and pepper

finely chopped red chillies, to garnish

1   Place the oil, ginger, garlic, shallots, turmeric, chillies, lemon grass and half of the coconut milk in a food processor and process until fairly smooth.

2   Heat a large nonstick wok and pour the coconut mixture into it. Stir-fry over a high heat for 3–4 minutes and then add the remaining coconut milk, the stock and lime leaves. Bring to the boil, then reduce the heat and simmer gently, uncovered, for 10 minutes.

3   Add the courgettes and baby sweetcorn to the mixture and simmer for 6–7 minutes. Stir in the tofu, soy sauce and lime juice, season to taste and cook gently for 1–2 minutes.

4   Remove from the heat and stir in the fresh coriander. Serve in bowls, garnished with chopped red chillies.

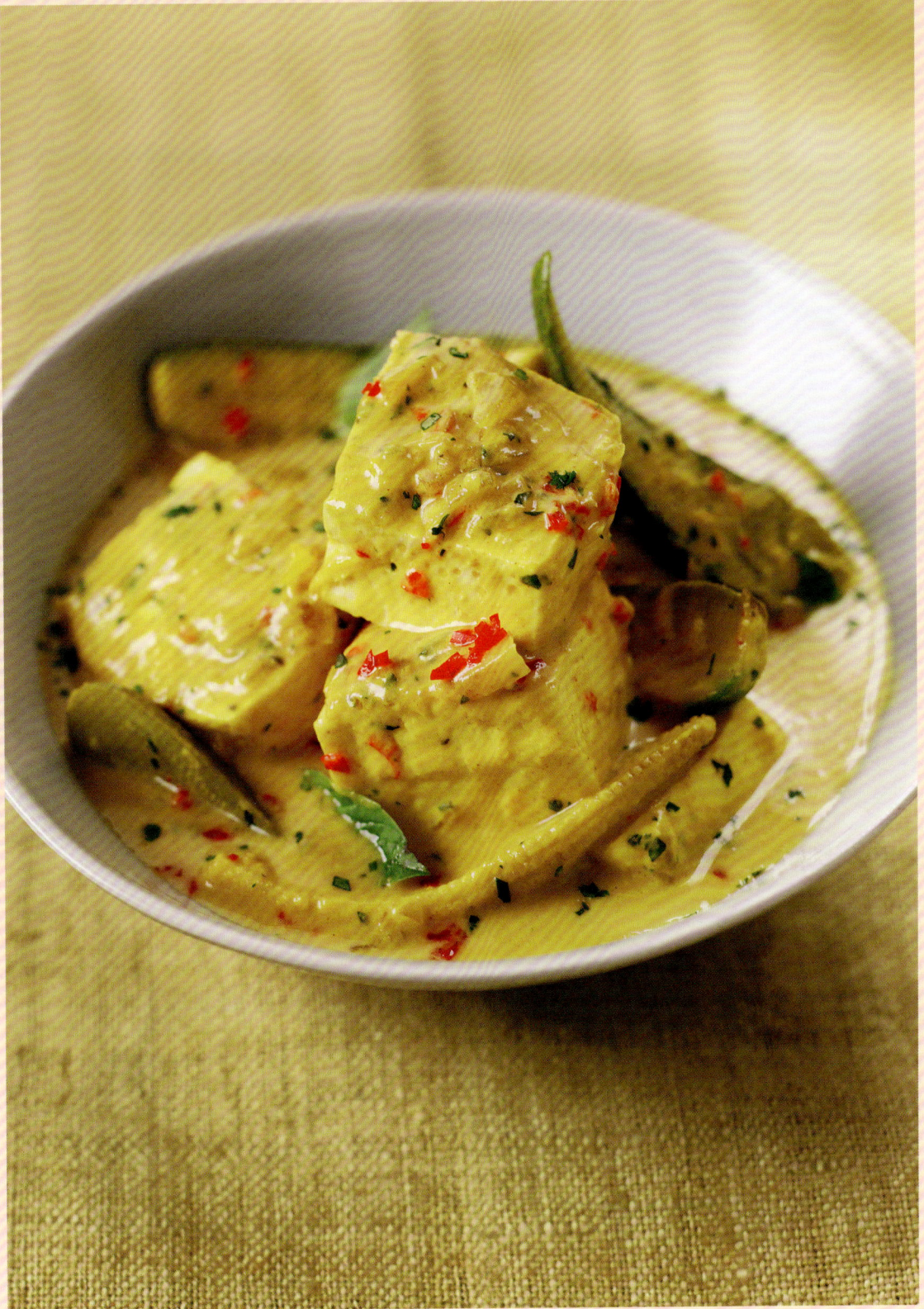

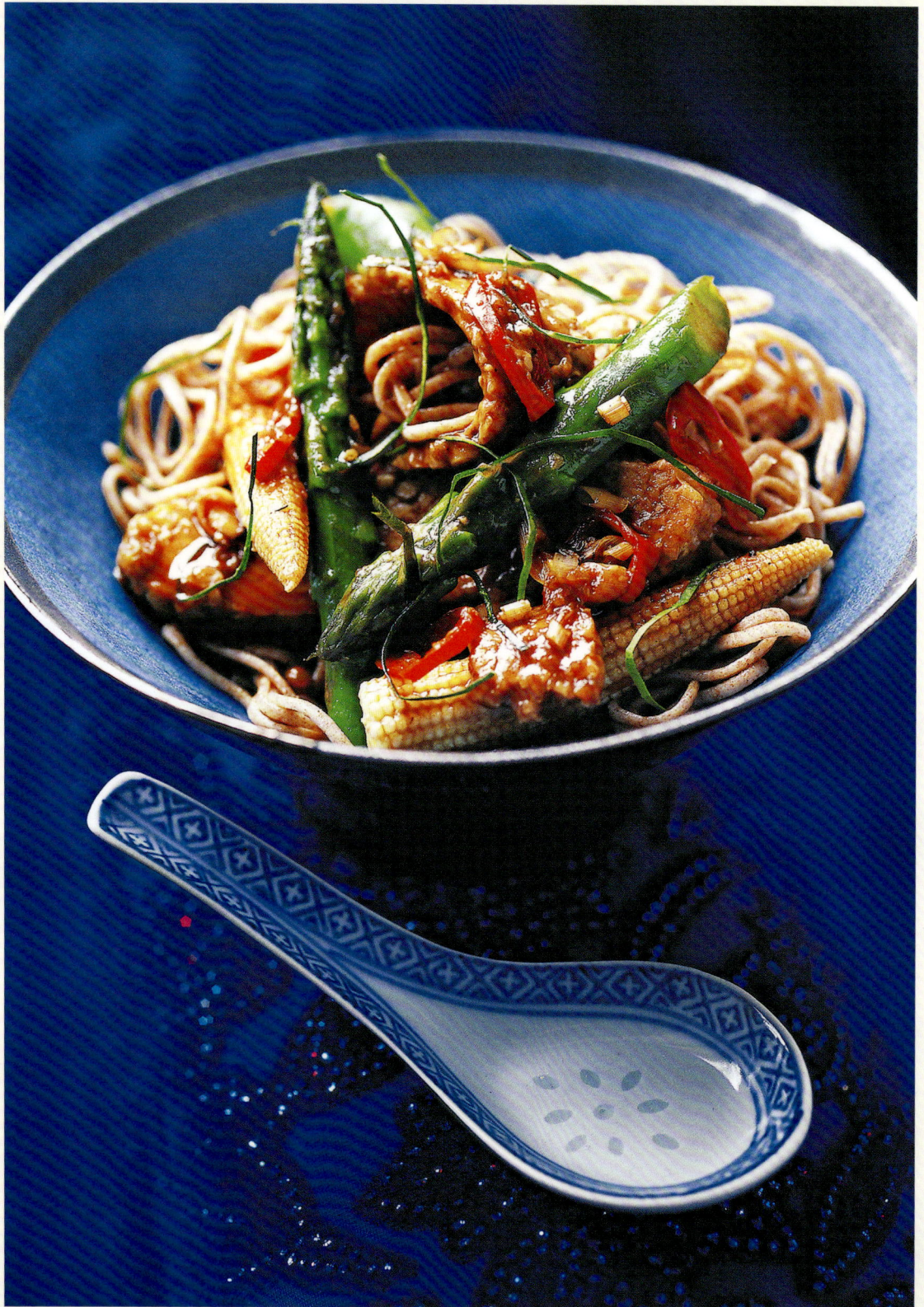

Spicy Tempeh & Vegetable Stir-fry

Mixing up your protein sources is a great way to keep things interesting. Tempeh is a plant-based ingredient made from fermented soybeans, but its protein profile rivals that of animal protein. Plus, the fermentation process makes it gut healthy.

SERVES 4

1 tablespoon olive oil

2 red chillies, sliced

2 lemon grass stalks, finely sliced

2 kaffir lime leaves

1 large garlic clove, crushed

1 tablespoon chopped fresh root ginger

1 tablespoon tamarind paste

2 tablespoons vegetable stock

2 teaspoons shoyu or tamari sauce

1 tablespoon clear honey

500 g (1 lb) tempeh or firm tofu, cut
    into strips

125 g (4 oz) baby sweetcorn

125 g (4 oz) asparagus spears, halved

1 Heat the oil in a wok over a high heat until the oil starts to shimmer. Add the chillies, lemon grass, lime leaves, garlic and ginger, then turn the heat down to medium and stir-fry for 2–3 minutes.

2 Add the tamarind paste, stock, shoyu or tamari sauce and honey and cook for 2–3 minutes until the sauce has become thick and glossy.

3 Add the tempeh, sweetcorn and asparagus and stir-fry for about 2 minutes to warm through, then serve.

tip | If you can't get your hands on tempeh, tofu works well here too!

Spinach & Tomato Dhal

Turmeric and ginger are anti-inflammatory superheroes, both shown to improve insulin resistance, a fundamental driver of many PCOS symptoms. Adding anti-inflammatory spices to a warming, hearty dhal dish is a great way to incorporate them into your diet, plus you can also add extra nutrient-dense dark leafy green vegetables like spinach.

SERVES 4

250 g (8 oz) dried red split lentils, rinsed and drained

½ teaspoon ground turmeric

2 green chillies, deseeded and chopped

2 teaspoons peeled and grated fresh root ginger

1 litre (1¾ pints) water

400 g (13 oz) can chopped tomatoes

250 g (8 oz) baby spinach leaves

salt

SPICED OIL

1 tablespoon olive oil

1 shallot, thinly sliced

12 curry leaves

1 teaspoon black mustard seeds

1 teaspoon cumin seeds

1 dried red chilli, broken into small pieces

1　Place the lentils in a large saucepan with the turmeric, chillies, ginger and measured water. Bring to the boil, then reduce the heat and simmer, uncovered, for 40 minutes, or until the lentils have broken down and the mixture has thickened.

2　Add the tomatoes and cook for a further 10 minutes, or until thickened. Stir in the spinach and cook for 2–3 minutes until wilted.

3　Prepare the spiced oil. Heat the oil in a small frying pan, add the shallot and cook over a medium-high heat, stirring, for 2–3 minutes until golden brown. Add all the remaining ingredients and cook, stirring constantly, for 1–2 minutes until the seeds start to pop.

4　Tip the spiced oil into the dhal, stir well and season to taste with salt. Serve with brown rice, if liked.

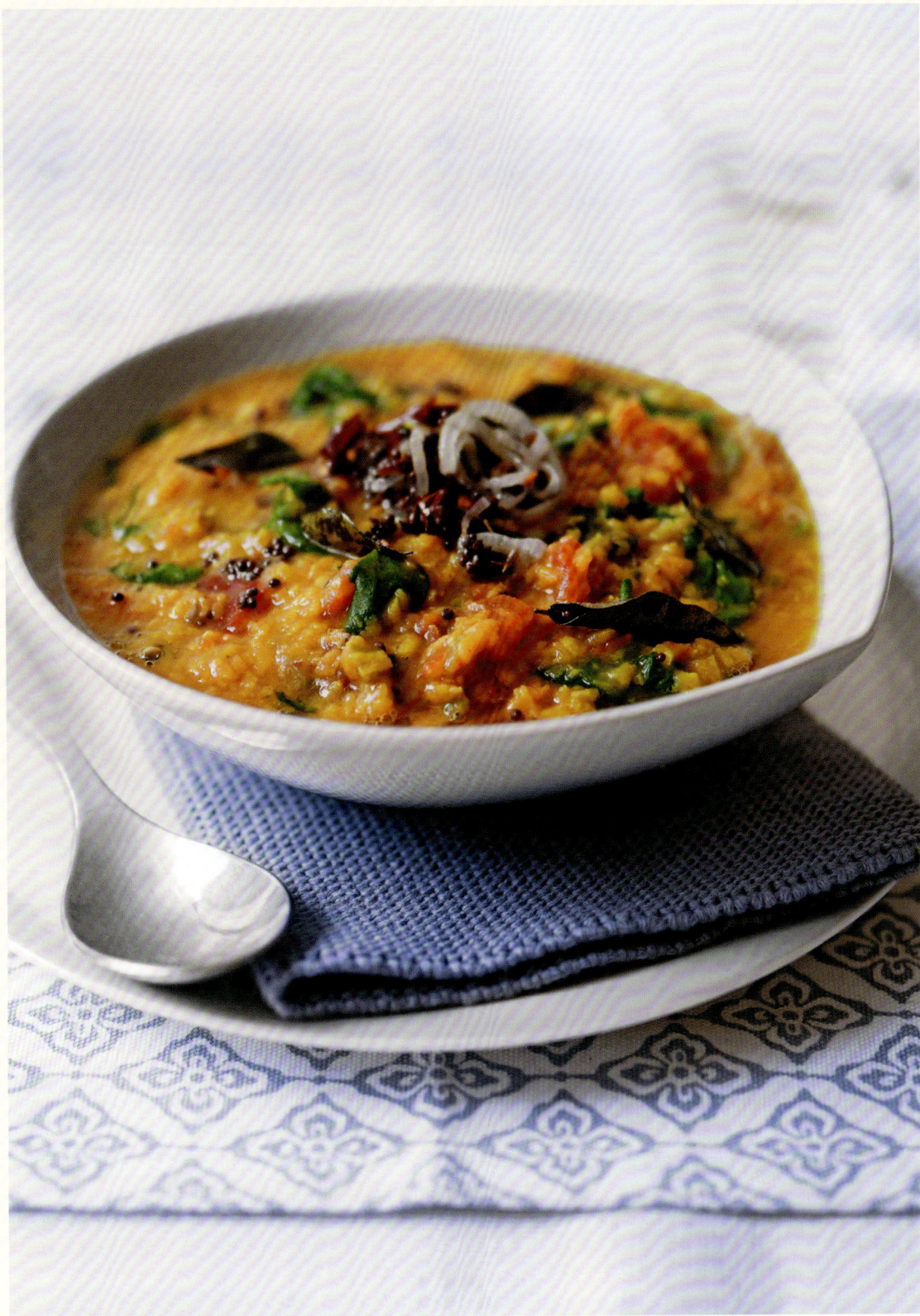

Spicy Tofu
with Pak Choi & Spring Onions

Curries are a great way to cram in a number of anti-inflammatory, PCOS-friendly spices such as turmeric and ginger. Curcumin, the active ingredient in turmeric, has been shown to help aid insulin resistance and reduce fasting blood sugar levels in those with PCOS. It can help to reduce oxidative stress in the body due to its antioxidant properties, potentially making it a useful spice in improving egg health and therefore, fertility outcomes.

SERVES 4

2 tablespoons olive oil

2 teaspoons grated fresh root ginger

8 garlic cloves, roughly chopped

4 shallots, finely chopped

2 red chillies, deseeded and chopped

8-cm (3-inch) length of trimmed
   lemon grass stalk, finely chopped

1 teaspoon ground turmeric

400 ml (14 fl oz) can coconut milk

200 ml (7 fl oz) hot vegetable stock

400 g (13 oz) baby pak choi, halved
   or quartered

200 g (7 oz) mangetout

400 g (14 oz) firm tofu, cubed

1 tablespoon dark soy sauce

1 tablespoon lime juice

6 spring onions, thinly sliced

salt and pepper

TO GARNISH

small handful of Thai basil leaves

sliced red chillies

1   Put the oil, ginger, garlic, shallots, chopped red chillies, lemon grass, turmeric and half of the coconut milk in a food processor or blender and blend until fairly smooth.

2   Heat a large nonstick wok or frying pan until hot, add the coconut milk mixture and stir-fry over a high heat for 3–4 minutes. Add the remaining coconut milk and the stock and bring to the boil, then reduce the heat to low and simmer gently, uncovered, for 6–8 minutes.

3   Add the pak choi, mangetout and tofu and simmer for a further 6–7 minutes. Stir in the soy sauce and lime juice, then season to taste and simmer for another 1–2 minutes.

4   Remove from the heat and stir in the spring onions. Ladle into warm bowls. Serve scattered with Thai basil leaves and sliced red chillies.

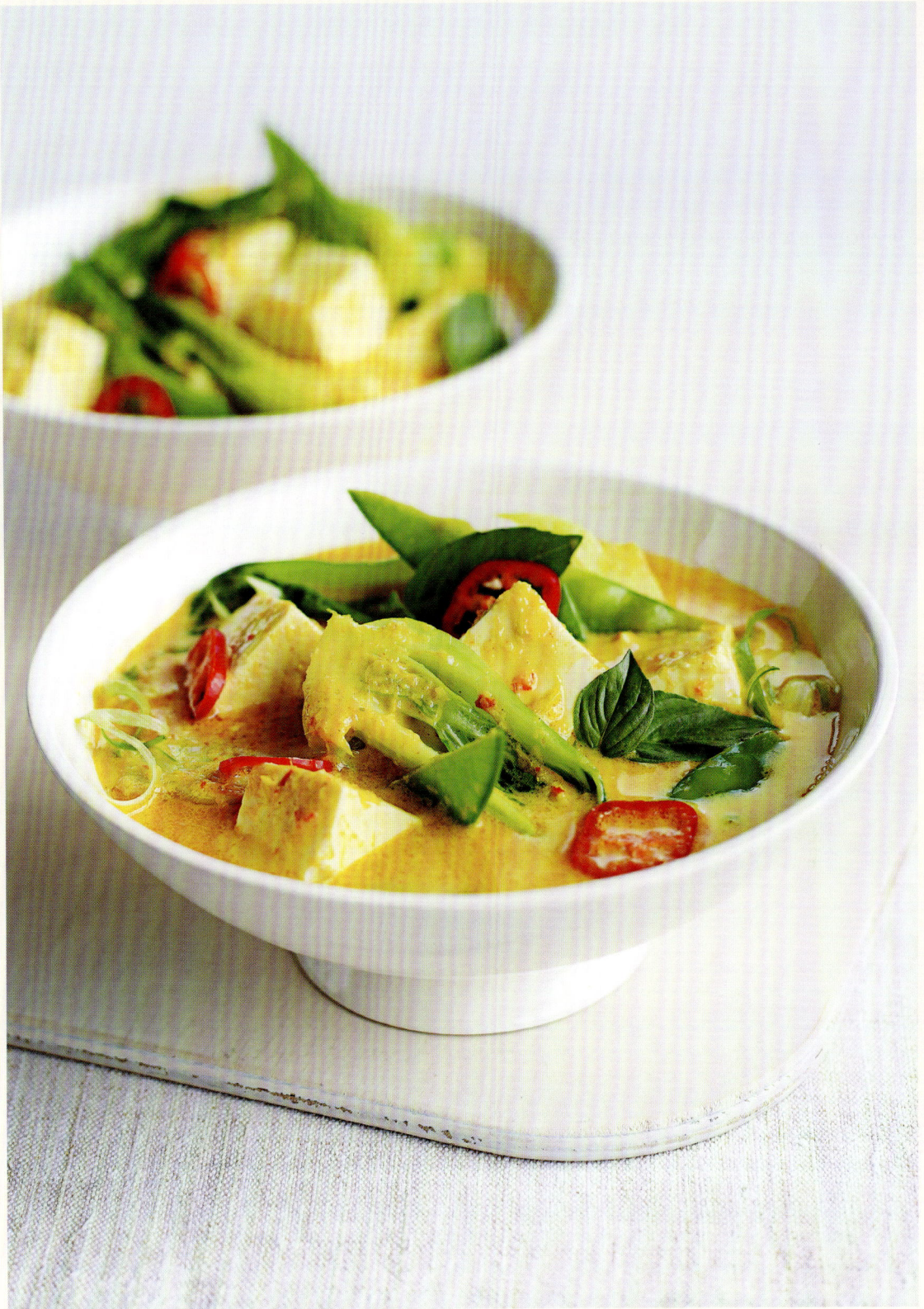

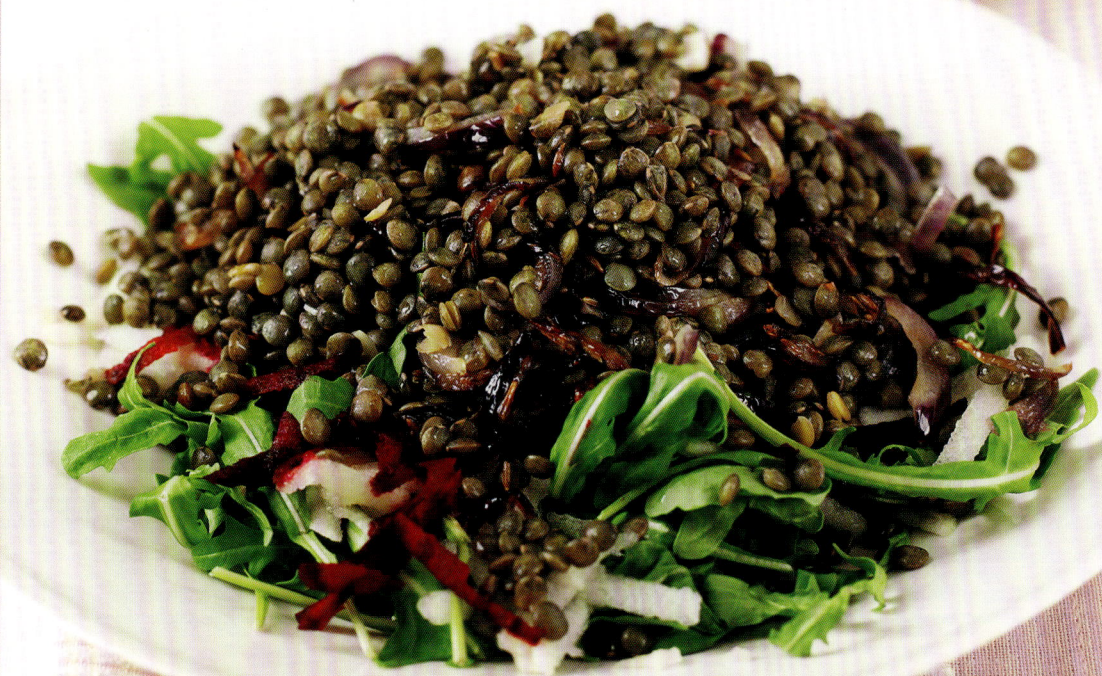

Cumin Lentils
with Yogurt Dressing

Sometimes, lentils can feel a bit tricky to incorporate into meals. While they are packed full of plant-based protein, fibre and a number of PCOS-friendly phytonutrients, it can be easy to avoid them if you aren't sure how to cook them well. This recipe is a great way of giving the humble lentil a bit of love with spices, fruit and veg. What's more, you don't even need to cook lentils from scratch, as most supermarkets offer great pre-cooked lentils, which you can heat up within a matter of minutes.

SERVES 4

4 tablespoons olive oil

2 red onions, thinly sliced

2 garlic cloves, chopped

2 teaspoon cumin seeds

500 g (1 lb) cooked Puy lentils

125 g (4 oz) peppery leaves, such as
    beetroot or rocket

1 large raw beetroot, peeled and
    coarsely grated

1 Granny Smith apple, peeled and
    coarsely grated (optional)

lemon juice, to serve

salt and pepper

YOGURT DRESSING

300 ml (½ pint) Greek yogurt

2 tablespoons lemon juice

½ teaspoon ground cumin

15 g (½ oz) mint leaves, chopped

1   Heat the oil in a frying pan and fry the red onions over a medium heat for about 8 minutes until soft and golden. Add the garlic and cumin seeds and cook for a further 5 minutes.

2   Mix the onion mixture into the lentils, season well and leave to cool.

3   Make the dressing by mixing together the ingredients in a small bowl.

4   Serve the cooled lentils on a bed of leaves, with the grated beetroot and apple, if liked, a couple of spoonfuls of minty yogurt dressing and a generous squeeze of lemon juice.

tip | Add some extra protein here if you need it, such as crumbled tofu or feta, salmon or chicken.

Spinach & Sweet Potato Cakes

Making the swap to complex carbohydrates might feel daunting, but having fun with how you prepare them can make maintaining a PCOS-healthy diet feel like a breeze. Sweet potato, the starchy base of these cakes, helps to keep energy and insulin levels stable, due to its fibre content.

SERVES 4

500 g (1 lb) sweet potatoes, peeled and
    cut into chunks
125 g (4 oz) spinach leaves
4–5 spring onions, finely sliced,
    plus extra to garnish
olive oil, for shallow-frying
3 tablespoons sesame seeds
4 tablespoons plain flour
salt and pepper
lime wedges, to serve

RED CHILLI & COCONUT DIP

200 ml (7 fl oz) coconut cream
2 red chillies, deseeded and finely
    chopped
1 lemon grass stalk, thinly sliced
3 kaffir lime leaves, shredded
small bunch of fresh coriander, chopped
2 tablespoons sesame oil

1 Cook the sweet potatoes in lightly salted boiling water for about 20 minutes or until tender. Drain, then return them to the pan and place over a low heat for a minute, stirring so the excess moisture evaporates. Lightly mash with a fork.

2 Meanwhile, put the spinach in a colander and pour over boiling water until wilted. Refresh in cold water and squeeze dry. Stir into the mash, then add the spring onions. Season well.

3 For the dip, gently warm the coconut cream in a pan with the chillies, lemon grass and lime leaves for 10 minutes. Don't let it boil. Set aside to infuse.

4 Heat the olive oil in a large pan. Use your hands to form the potato mixture into 12 cakes. Mix together the sesame seeds and flour and sprinkle over the cakes, then carefully lower them into the oil and fry in batches until golden and crispy. Drain on kitchen paper and keep warm while you cook the rest.

5 Stir the coriander and sesame oil into the dip and serve with the potato cakes, with lime wedges and spring onions.

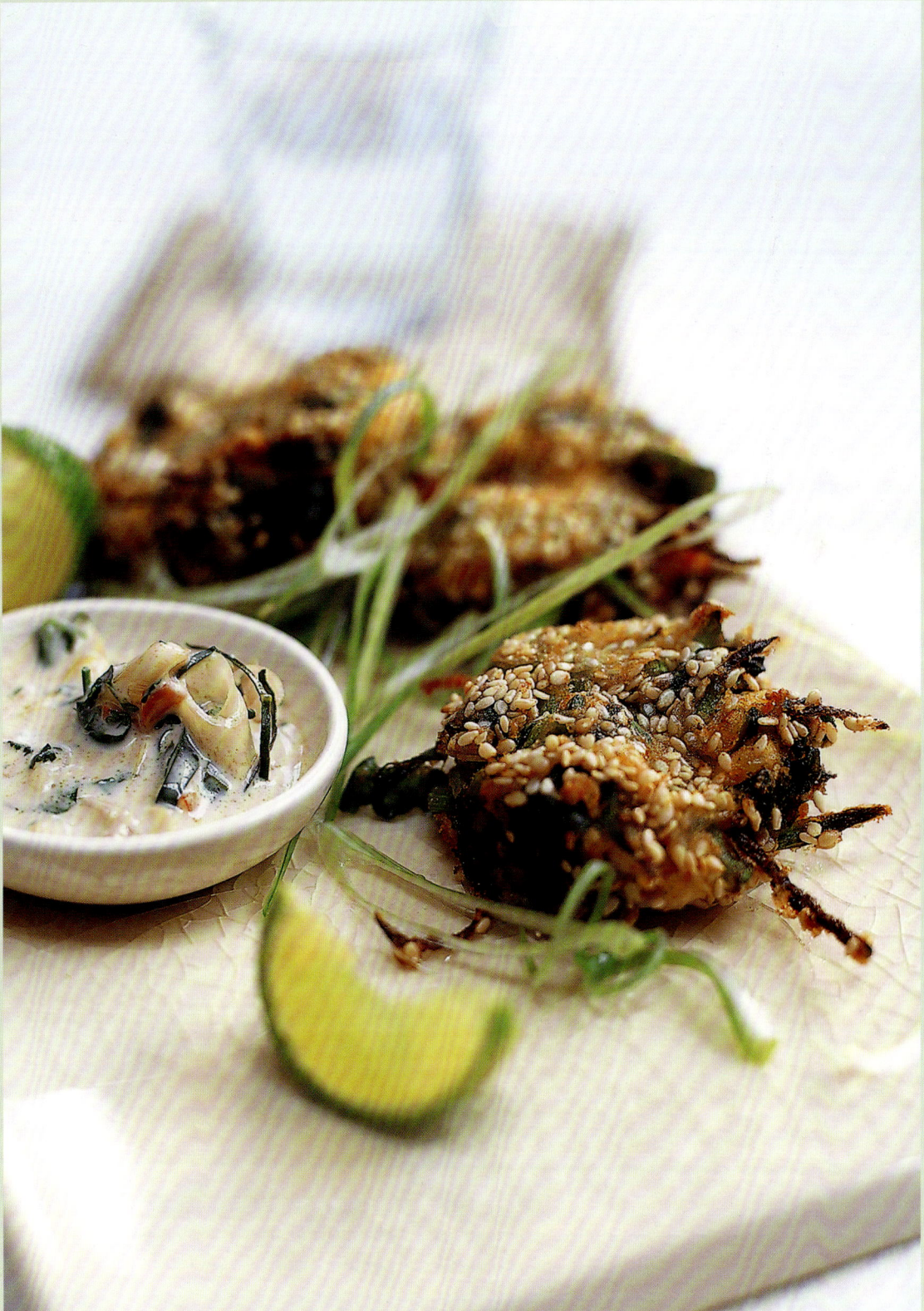

Spicy Courgette Fritters

Good low-carb, high-protein lunches can be hard to come by, but these courgette fritters make for the perfect choice if you're looking for something a little different. Not only are courgettes high in fibre, keeping you fuller for longer and blood sugar levels stable, but they also contain a number of micronutrients including vitamin C, vitamin A and folate.

SERVES **4**

3 courgettes
2 large spring onions, grated
1 garlic clove, finely chopped
finely grated zest of 1 lemon
4 tablespoons gram flour
2 teaspoons medium curry powder
1 fresh red chilli, deseeded and
    finely chopped
2 tablespoons finely chopped
    mint leaves
2 tablespoons finely chopped
    coriander leaves
2 eggs, lightly beaten
2 tablespoons light olive oil
salt and pepper

1   Grate the courgettes into a colander. Sprinkle lightly with salt and leave for at least 1 hour to drain. Squeeze out the remaining liquid.

2   Place the remaining ingredients, except the eggs and olive oil, in a mixing bowl and add the courgettes. Season lightly, bearing in mind you have already salted the courgettes, and mix well. Add the eggs and mix again to combine.

3   Heat half of the olive oil in a large frying pan over a medium-high heat. Place dessertspoonfuls of the mixture, well spaced, in the pan and press down with the back of the spoon. Cook for 1–2 minutes on each side until golden and cooked through. Remove from the pan and keep warm. Repeat to cook the rest of the fritters in the same way, adding the remaining oil to the pan when necessary.

tip   Boost the protein by adding a couple of eggs on top of your fritters. Or, if eggs aren't your thing, a side of Greek yogurt makes a perfect dip.

Lime & Ginger Chicken Bowl

A zesty, flavourful and nutritious lunch bowl. Using ginger in your meals is a great way to introduce a different, exciting flavour profile, plus it is also highly beneficial for our health. Ginger is anti-inflammatory, reducing and even inhibiting the production of inflammatory mediators. It's also a great one for digestive ailments, supporting motility, and reducing bloating and abdominal pain.

SERVES **2**

200 g (7 oz) chicken breast, sliced

175 g (6 oz) brown rice

125 g (4 oz) mangetout (optional)

salt

lime wedges, to serve

MARINADE

1 tablespoon olive oil

2 tablespoons light soy sauce

2.5-cm (1-inch) piece of fresh root ginger, peeled and grated

1 garlic clove, peeled and grated

DRESSING

2.5-cm (1-inch) piece of fresh root ginger, peeled and grated

grated zest and juice of 2 limes

2 tablespoons light soy sauce

2 tablespoons vegetable oil

1 bunch of coriander, chopped

1 Mix the chicken with the marinade ingredients and leave in the refrigerator to marinate for about 15 minutes.

2 Cook the rice in a large pan of lightly salted boiling water according to the packet instructions until just tender. Drain well and set aside to cool slightly.

3 Meanwhile, combine the dressing ingredients and set aside.

4 Place the mangetout in a small bowl with enough boiling water to cover. Set aside for 2–3 minutes until they are just tender but still have a slight crunch, then drain and set aside.

5 Heat a dry frying pan and cook the marinated chicken gently for 10–12 minutes, stirring occasionally, until cooked through but not browned.

6 Meanwhile, stir the dressing into the rice. Fold through the cooked chicken and mangetout and spoon into dishes. Serve with lime wedges, for squeezing.

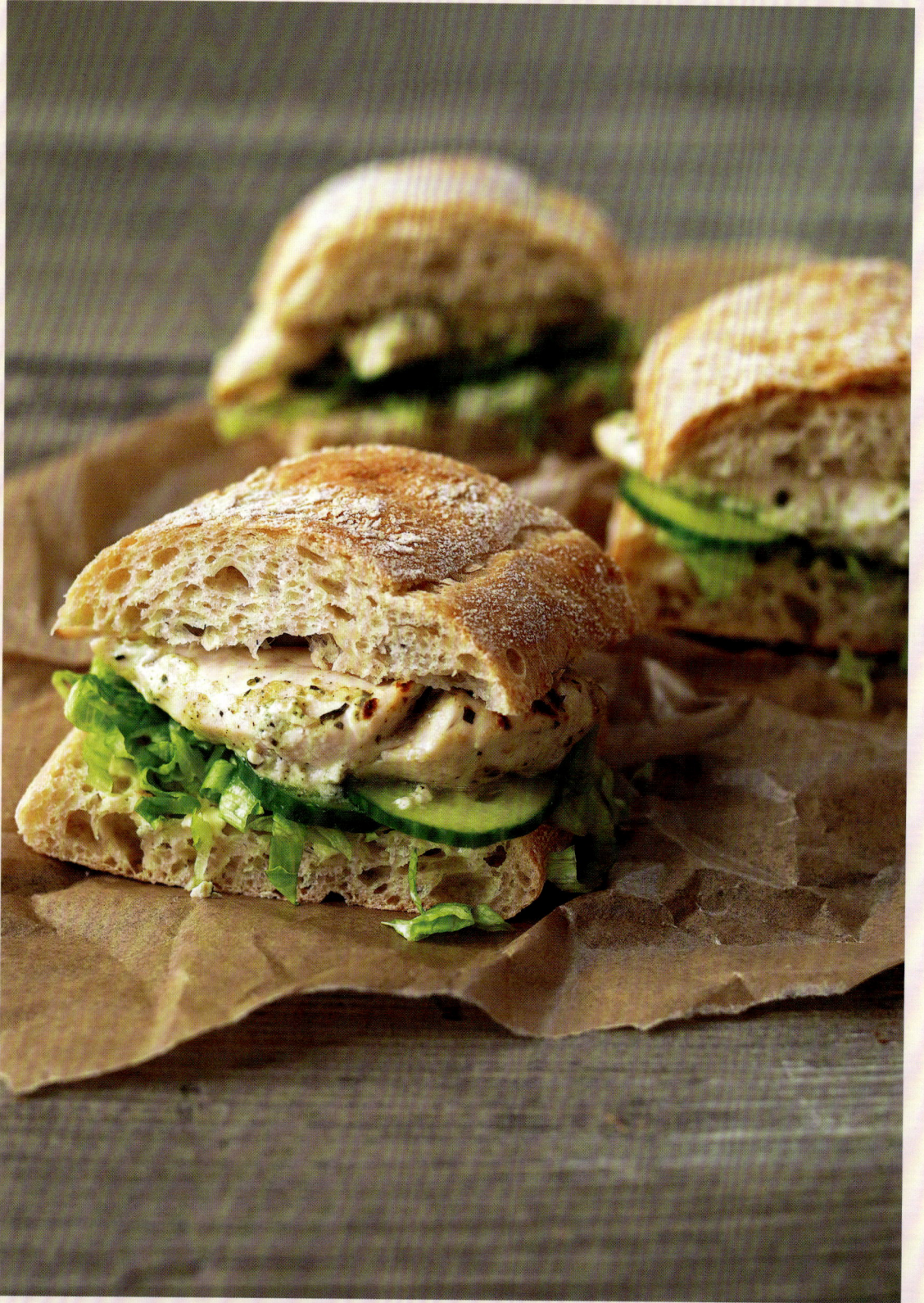

Thai-style Grilled Chicken Sandwich

How to make a sandwich PCOS-friendly? Include a source of protein, fat and extra fibre in between wholegrain or sourdough bread. This helps to keep blood sugar levels stable, preventing dips later on in the afternoon.

SERVES **2**

200 g (7 oz) mini chicken fillets
1 tablespoon Thai red or green curry paste
2 tablespoons natural yogurt

TO SERVE

1 tablespoon natural yogurt
1 sourdough ciabatta roll, split lengthways
small handful of shredded Iceberg or
     romaine lettuce
¼ cucumber, sliced

1   Place the chicken fillets in a bowl with the curry paste and yogurt. Mix together to combine, then arrange on the rack of a foil-lined grill tray and slide under a preheated medium-hot grill. Grill for 7–8 minutes, turning once, until cooked through and lightly charred.

2   To build the sandwich, spread the yogurt inside the sourdough roll and top with the lettuce and sliced cucumber. Add the cooked chicken fillets, then cut into 4 to serve.

tip | Add some avocado for a source of healthy fats.

Chicken Burgers
with Tomato Salsa

Chicken mince is a great protein to play around with in your PCOS-friendly recipes, often packing in around 30 g (1¼ oz) of protein per 125 g (4 oz) mince!

SERVES 4

1 garlic clove, crushed

3 spring onions, finely sliced

1 tablespoon pesto

2 tablespoons chopped mixed herbs,
   such as parsley, tarragon and thyme

375 g (12 oz) minced chicken

2 sun-dried tomatoes, finely chopped

1 teaspoon olive oil

TOMATO SALSA

250 g (8 oz) cherry tomatoes, quartered

1 red chilli, deseeded and finely chopped

1 tablespoon chopped coriander

grated zest and juice of 1 lime

TO SERVE

toasted wholemeal burger bun

mixed salad leaves

1   Mix together all the burger ingredients, except the oil, in a bowl. Divide the mixture into 4 and form into burgers. Cover and chill for 30 minutes.

2   Meanwhile, combine all the salsa ingredients in a bowl.

3   Brush the burgers with oil and cook under a preheated hot grill or on a barbecue for about 3–4 minutes on each side until cooked through.

4   Serve each burger in a toasted burger bun with the tomato salsa and salad leaves.

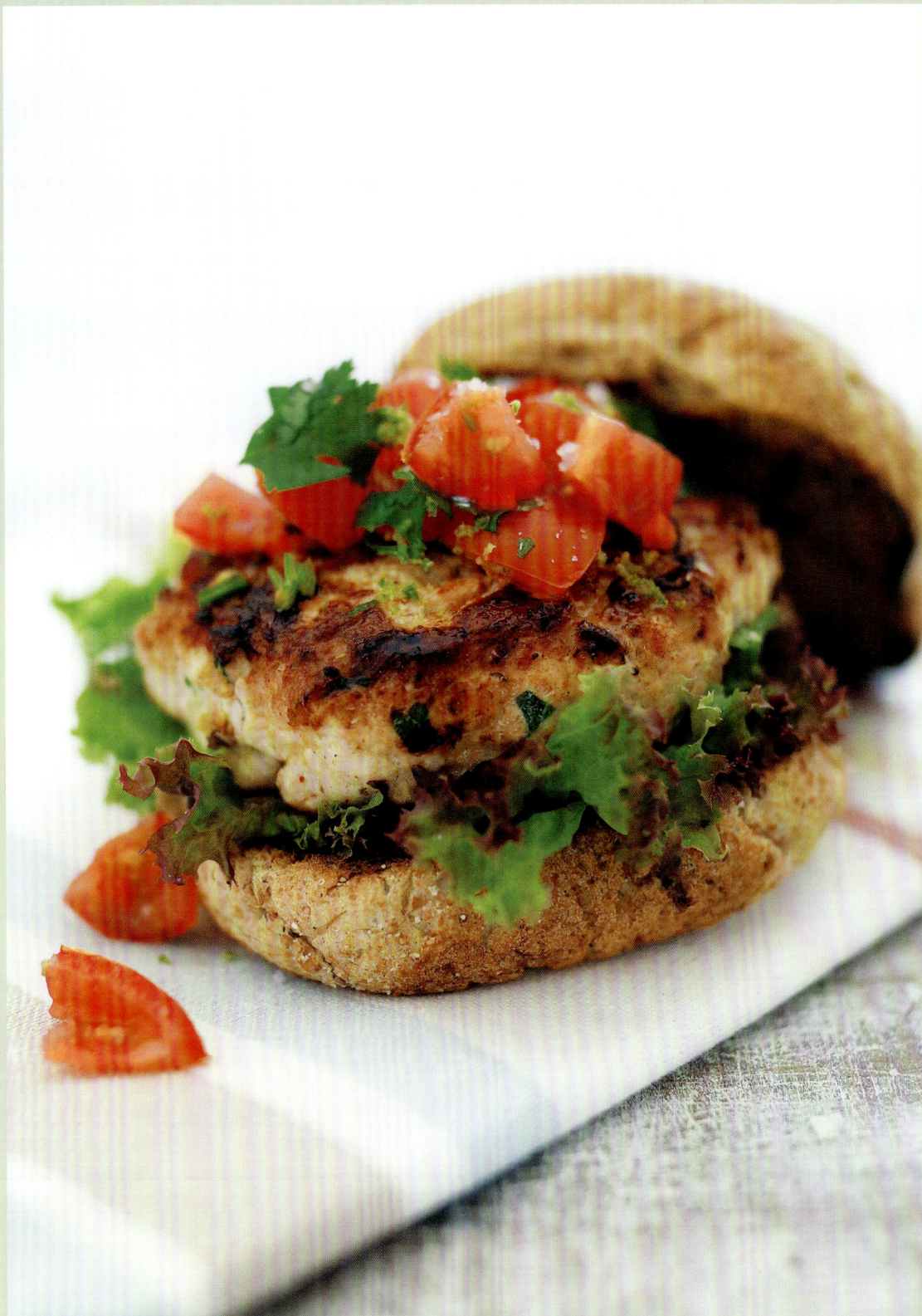

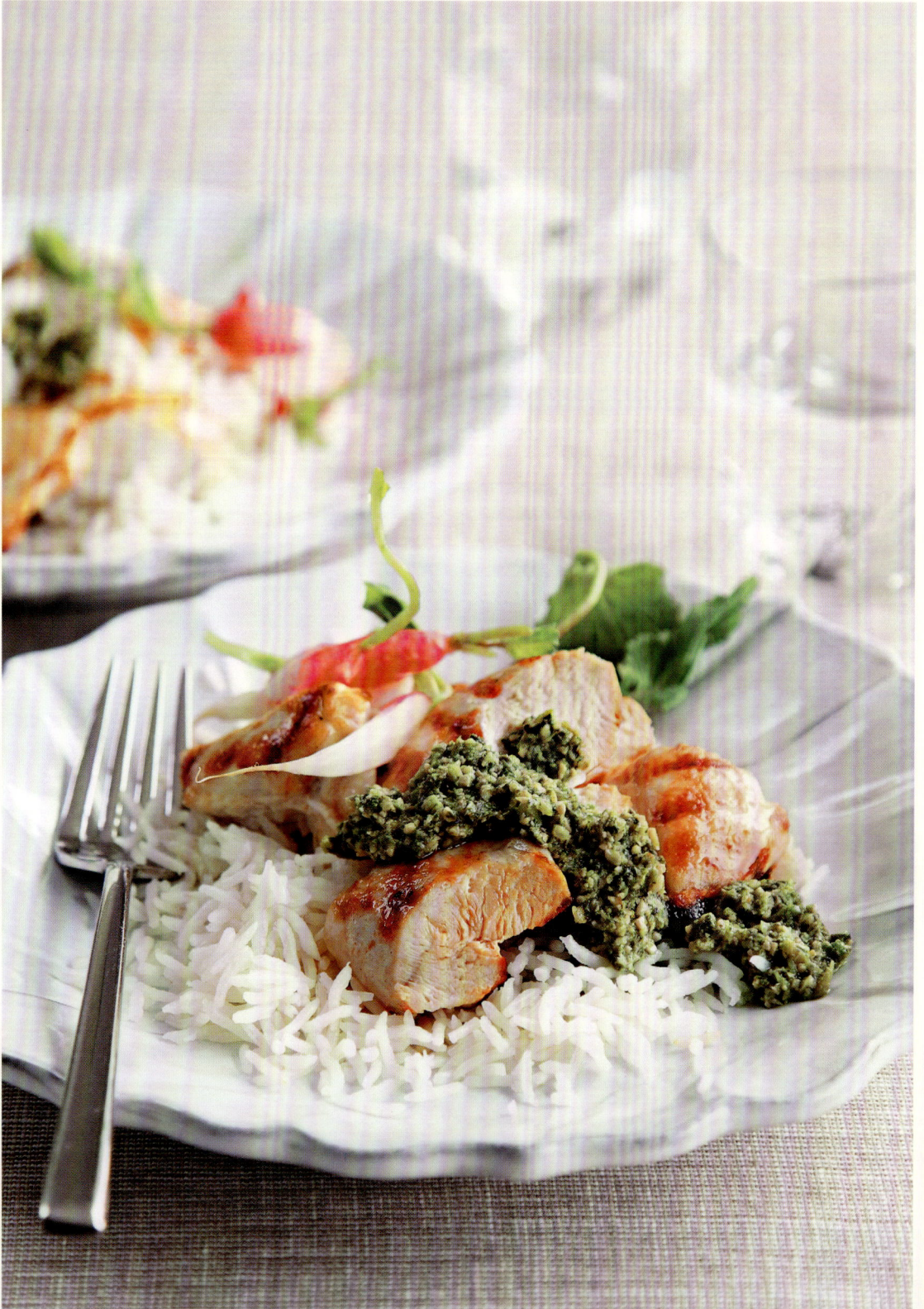

Chicken
with a Pumpkin Seed Sauce

Pumpkin seeds are rich in zinc, a key mineral for those with PCOS as it can help to regulate testosterone and reduce androgenic symptoms such as acne and excess hair growth. It also supports healthy thyroid function. Using pumpkin seeds as the base of a herby sauce is a great way to incorporate them into your meals.

SERVES 4

75 g (3 oz) pumpkin seeds

1 small onion, chopped

1 green chilli, deseeded, if liked, and chopped

½ teaspoon dried oregano

large handful of coriander leaves, including the stalks

200 ml (7 fl oz) chicken stock

2 tablespoons olive oil

4 skinless, boneless chicken breasts, about 125 g (4 oz) each

salt and pepper

TO SERVE

cooked rice

handful of sliced radishes

1 Heat a large, dry nonstick frying pan until hot, add the pumpkin seeds and dry-fry for 3–5 minutes, stirring frequently, until golden and starting to pop. Leave to cool.

2 When cool, place the pumpkin seeds in a food processor or blender with the onion, chilli, oregano, coriander and 75 ml (3 fl oz) of the stock and whizz to a smooth paste.

3 Heat 1 tablespoon of the oil in a saucepan, add the paste and cook for about 10 minutes, stirring frequently, until thickened. Pour in the remaining stock and simmer for 15 minutes.

4 Meanwhile, rub the remaining oil over the chicken, then season. Heat a griddle pan until smoking hot, add the chicken and cook for 5–7 minutes on each side until just cooked through. Cut into slices and arrange on a serving plate with cooked rice and some sliced radishes. Serve with the sauce spooned over.

Minced Beef
with Scrambled Eggs

Red meat gets a bit of a bad rep! However, the quality of that meat is key. Avoiding processed meat is important for all aspects of our health, but lean beef mince can be a great and easy way to top up key minerals and vitamins, all of which are supportive of our hormones. This lunch recipe is high in protein, keeping blood sugar levels stable all afternoon long and, as a result, preventing those dreaded mid-afternoon crashes.

SERVES 4

300 g (10 oz) minced beef

1½ tablespoons light soy sauce

3 teaspoons sesame oil

1 tablespoon Chinese rice wine or
    dry sherry

½ teaspoon salt

3 tablespoons groundnut oil

1 red onion, cut into thin wedges

1 red chilli, deseeded and finely chopped

3 eggs

black pepper

handful of coriander leaves, to garnish

cooked rice, to serve (optional)

1   Break up the beef with a fork and place it in a bowl with 1 tablespoon of the soy sauce, 2 teaspoons of the sesame oil and the rice wine. Stir in the salt and season with a generous grinding of black pepper. Leave to marinate for 15 minutes.

2   Heat 2 tablespoons of the groundnut oil in a wok over a high heat until the oil starts to shimmer. Add the onion and chilli and stir-fry for 2 minutes until it begins to colour. Add the beef and let the meat cook until it becomes golden but not browned. Drain in a sieve.

3   Wipe the wok clean, return it to the heat and pour in the remaining groundnut oil. While it heats up again, combine the eggs, remaining soy sauce and sesame oil and season lightly with freshly ground black pepper. Tip the mixture into the hot oil and scramble for about 1 minute until mostly set, but still moist and creamy. Return the cooked beef to the wok and stir-fry for 1 minute. Scatter with coriander and serve with rice, if liked.

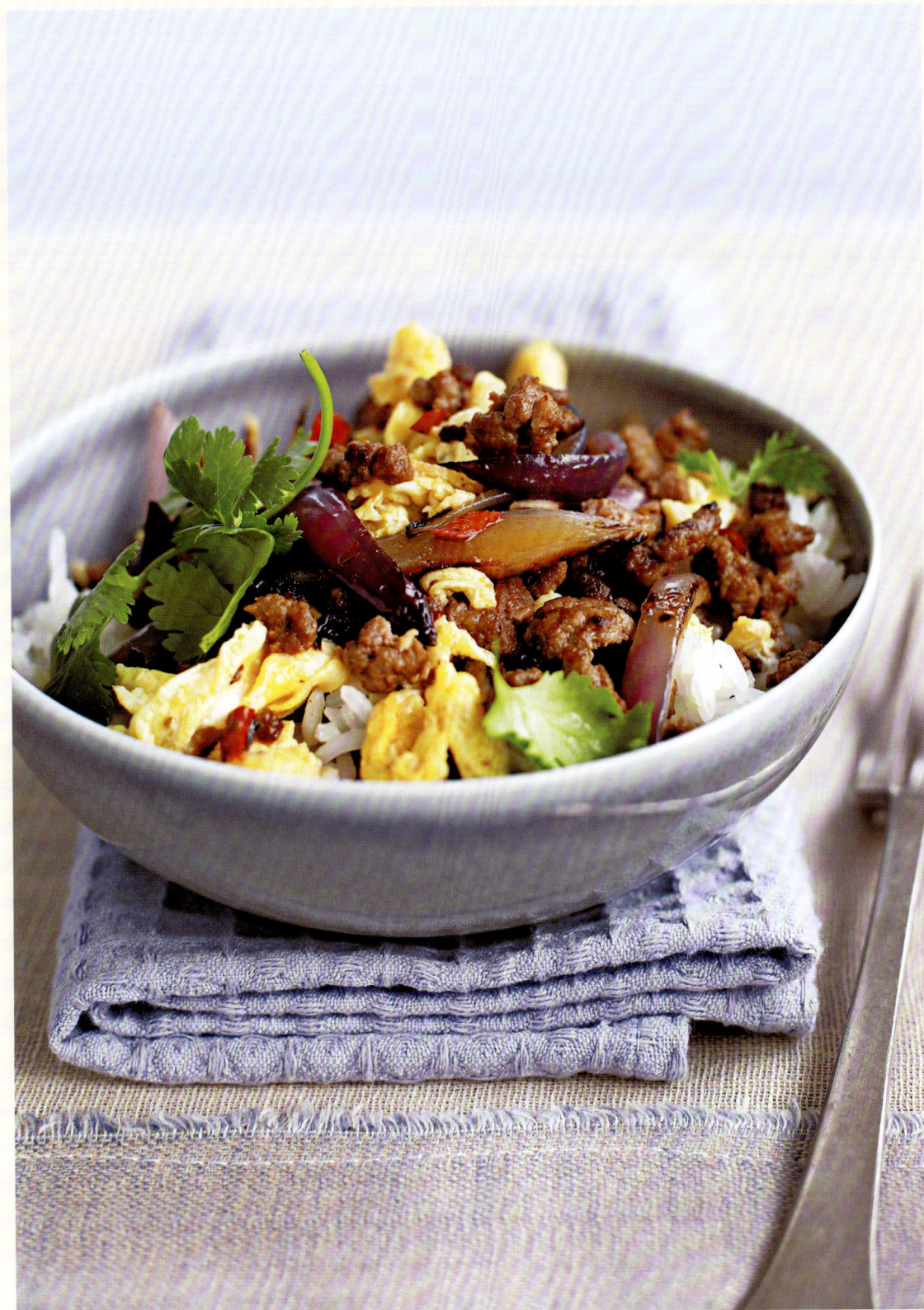

Spicy Grilled Sardines

When thinking about foods that are high in calcium, sardines might not be the first that comes to mind. However, due to their small, soft bones, they really do hold their own. Calcium, of course, is a key mineral for bone and muscle health, but it also supports a balanced mood as it plays an important role in regulating serotonin activity.

SERVES **2**

6 large prepared fresh sardines
1 teaspoon chopped garlic
finely grated zest and juice of ½ lemon
1 teaspoon ground cumin
1 teaspoon hot smoked paprika
1 tablespoon olive oil
salt and pepper

TO SERVE

crisp green salad
lemon halves
sourdough bread, toasted

1   Use a sharp knife to make 3 slashes on each side of the fish, cutting through the skin and flesh to the bone. Arrange the sardines on a baking sheet.

2   Mix together all the remaining ingredients, season to taste, then rub all over the fish to coat thoroughly.

3   Cook the sardines under a preheated hot grill or on a barbecue, turning once, for 3–5 minutes, or until cooked through. Serve with a crisp green salad, lemon halves and toasted sourdough.

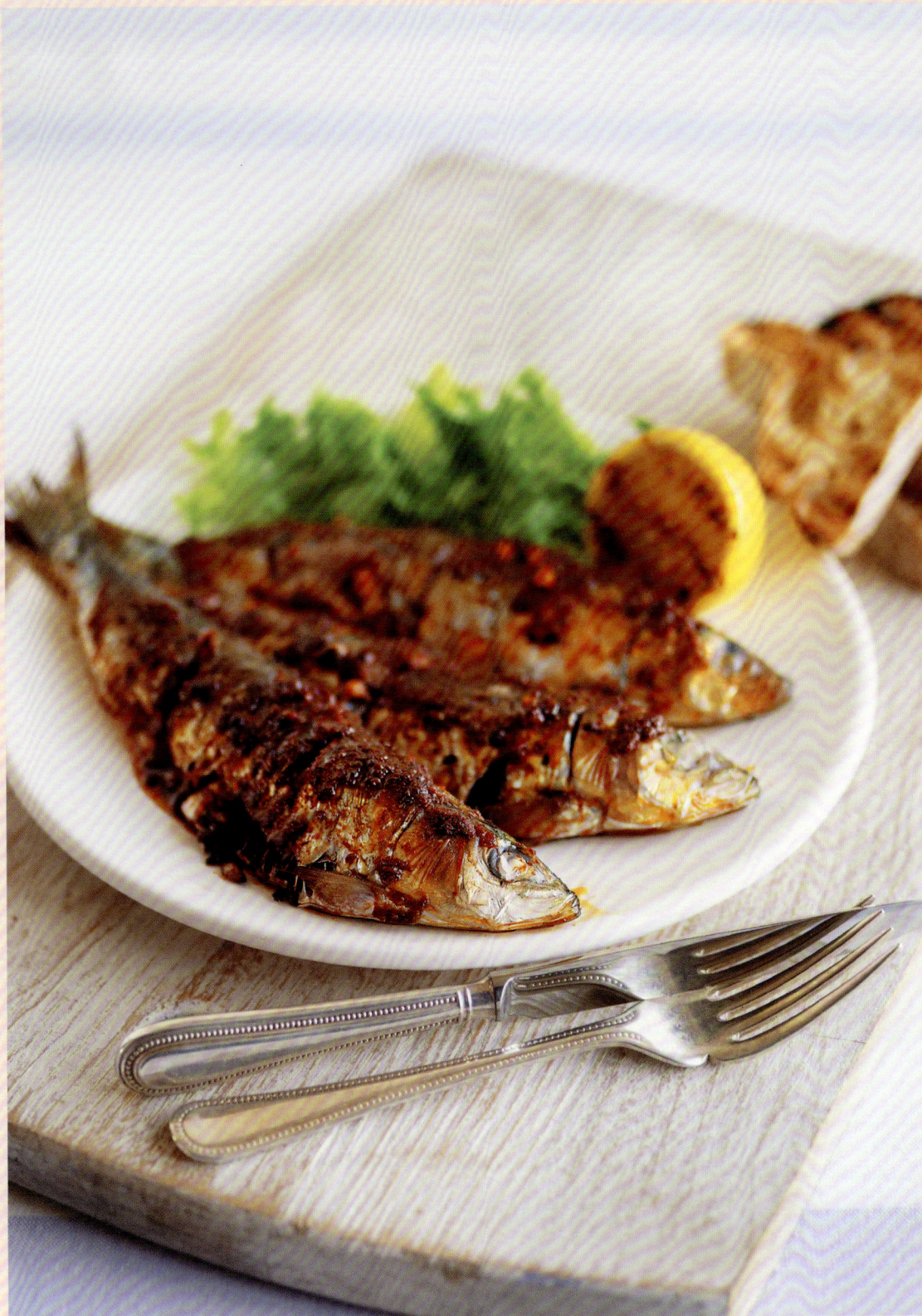

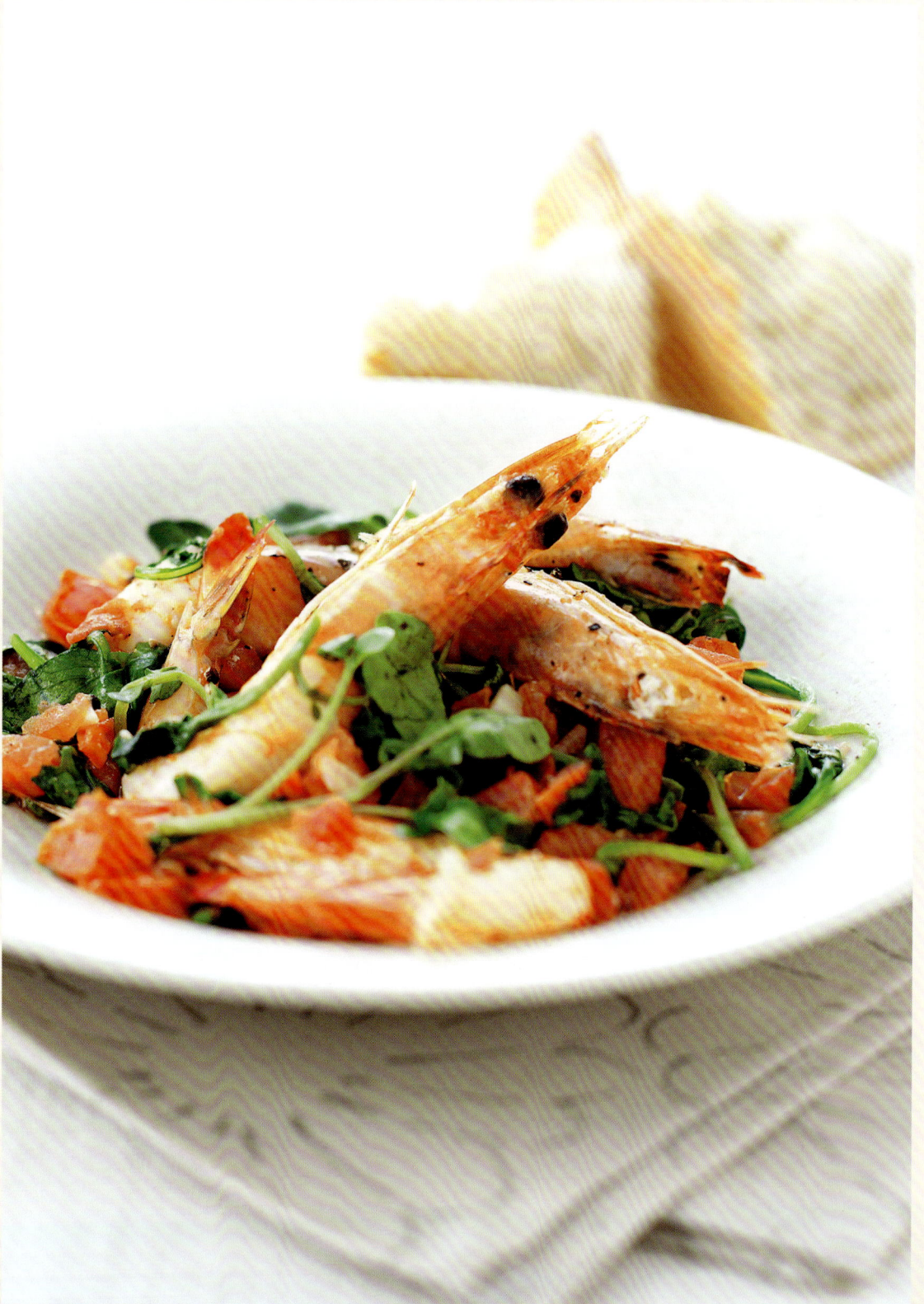

Prawns
with Green Leaves

Prawns are small but mighty, packing a good amount of protein in. They are also a quick source of protein, taking only a few minutes to cook. This recipe incorporates dark leafy greens alongside the prawns, which are also incredibly nutrient-dense, containing minerals such as magnesium and zinc, and vitamins C and folate.

SERVES **4**

1 tablespoon olive oil

20 large raw king prawns,
    with shells intact

1 garlic clove, chopped

125 g (4 oz) plum tomatoes, chopped

50 g (2 oz) rocket

50 g (2 oz) spinach leaves,
    tough stalks removed

50 g (2 oz) watercress,
    tough stalks removed

1 tablespoon lemon juice

salt and pepper

sourdough bread, to serve (optional)

1 Heat the oil in a large saucepan over a medium-high heat, add the prawns and garlic and season to taste. Cover tightly and cook, shaking the pan from time to time, for about 3 minutes, or until the prawns are cooked.

2 Add the tomatoes, rocket, spinach and watercress and stir until wilted. Squeeze over the lemon juice and check the seasoning.

3 Serve immediately, with sourdough bread if liked.

Lime & Coriander Sea Bass

White fish, like sea bass, is a super versatile protein due to its mild flavour, allowing you to get creative with seasoning. Sea bass contains a good amount of the mineral selenium, which helps to maintain healthy thyroid function and aids antioxidant status in the body. Add a portion of dark leafy greens or colourful veggies on the side, along with an optional portion of wholegrains, such as quinoa, and you have a perfectly balanced PCOS-friendly midweek lunch.

SERVES 4

150 g (5 oz) butter, softened

3 tablespoons chopped coriander, plus extra sprigs

1 large red chilli, deseeded and finely chopped

2 limes, zested and sliced

4 whole sea bass, gutted and scaled

2 tablespoons vegetable oil

salt and pepper

1   Mix together the butter, chopped coriander, chilli and lime zest. Season with salt and pepper. Spoon the butter mixture on to a sheet of clingfilm and roll it up to form a sausage. Twist the ends to enclose the butter and place it in the refrigerator to set.

2   Take the fish and make 3 slits in the flesh on each side. Slice the limes and place a few slices in the cavity of each fish, along with some coriander sprigs. Brush the outside of the fish lightly with the oil and season both sides generously with salt and pepper.

3   Place the fish either in a fish grill or directly on the rack of a medium-hot barbecue. Cook for 5 minutes on each side. The best way to test if the fish is cooked is by looking inside the cavity to see if the flesh has become opaque or if the fish is firm to the touch.

4   Slice the butter thinly into rounds, place into the cuts on the side of the fish and let it melt. Serve with a green salad.

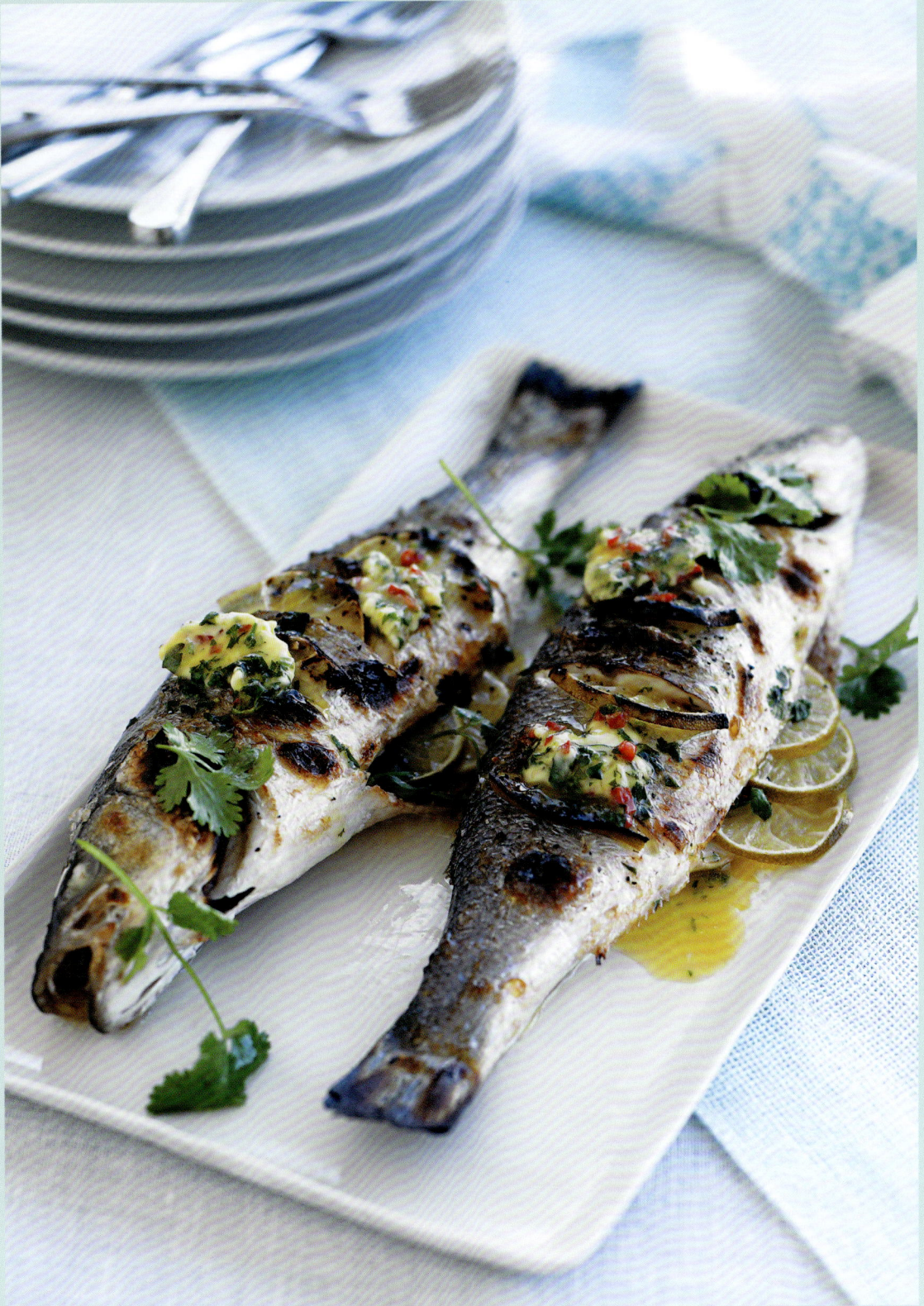

Mackerel
with Avocado Salsa

Gone are the days of fearing fat, especially when it comes to maintaining a healthy weight. Instead, embracing healthy fat helps to keep you full and support optimal hormone levels. This mackerel recipe is a great one for mid-week evenings when you just want something quick. It contains both monounsaturated fat from the avocado, and polyunsaturated fat, specifically omega-3, from the mackerel, shown to improve androgen levels in PCOS.

SERVES 4

8 mackerel fillets
2 lemons, plus extra wedges to serve
salt and pepper

AVOCADO SALSA

2 avocados, peeled, stoned and
    finely diced
zest and juice of 1 lime
1 red onion, finely chopped
½ cucumber, finely diced
1 handful of coriander leaves,
    finely chopped

1   Make 3 diagonal slashes across each mackerel fillet on the skin side and season well with salt and pepper. Cut the lemons in half, then squeeze the juice over the fish.

2   Lay on a grill rack, skin-side up, and cook under a preheated hot grill for 6–8 minutes, or until the skin is lightly charred and the flesh is just cooked through.

3   Meanwhile, to make the salsa, mix together the avocados and lime zest and juice, then add the onion, cucumber and most of the coriander (keep a little for serving). Toss well to mix and season to taste with salt and pepper.

4   Serve the mackerel hot, sprinkled with the remaining coriander, with the avocado salsa on the side and lemon wedges for squeezing over.

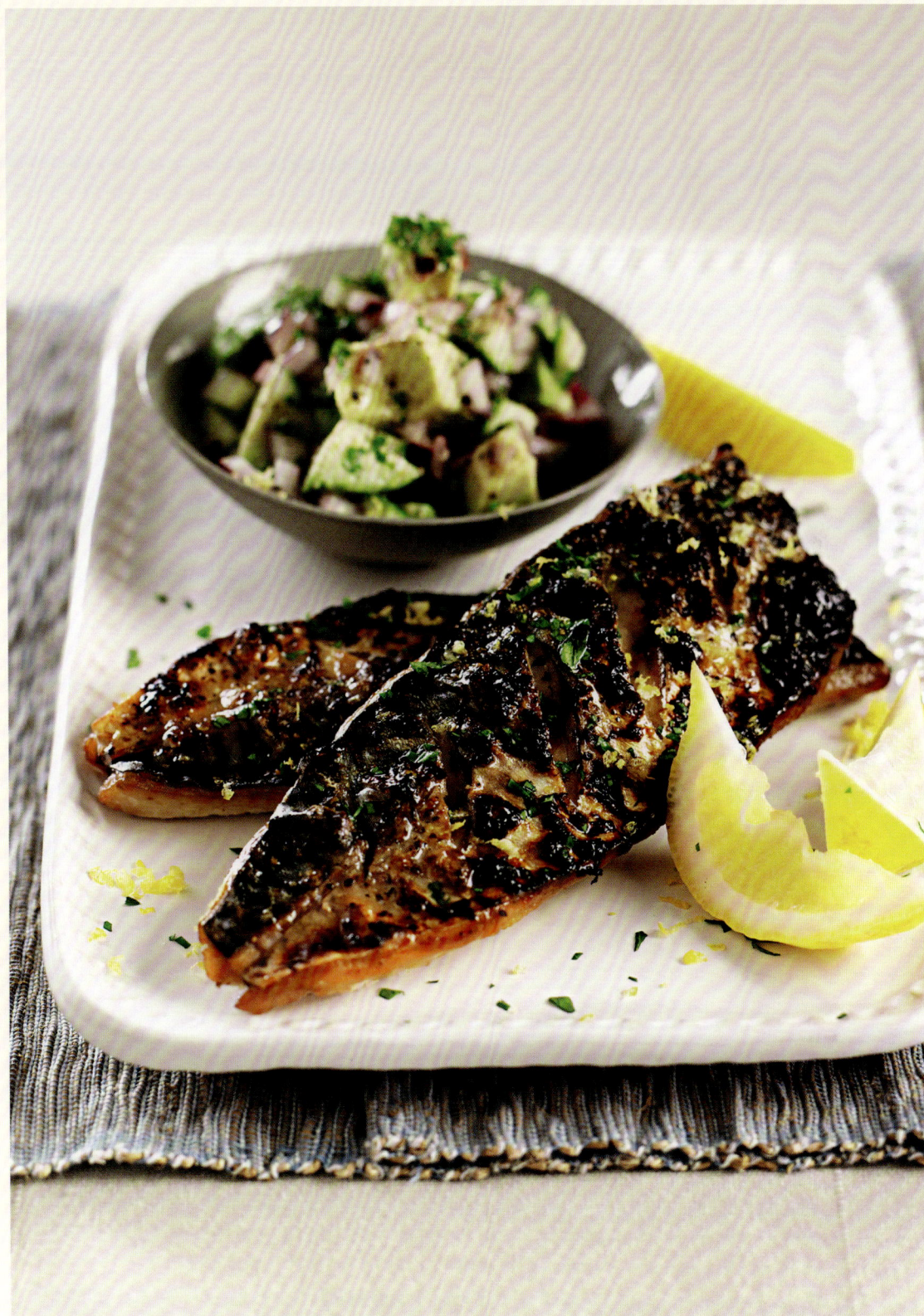

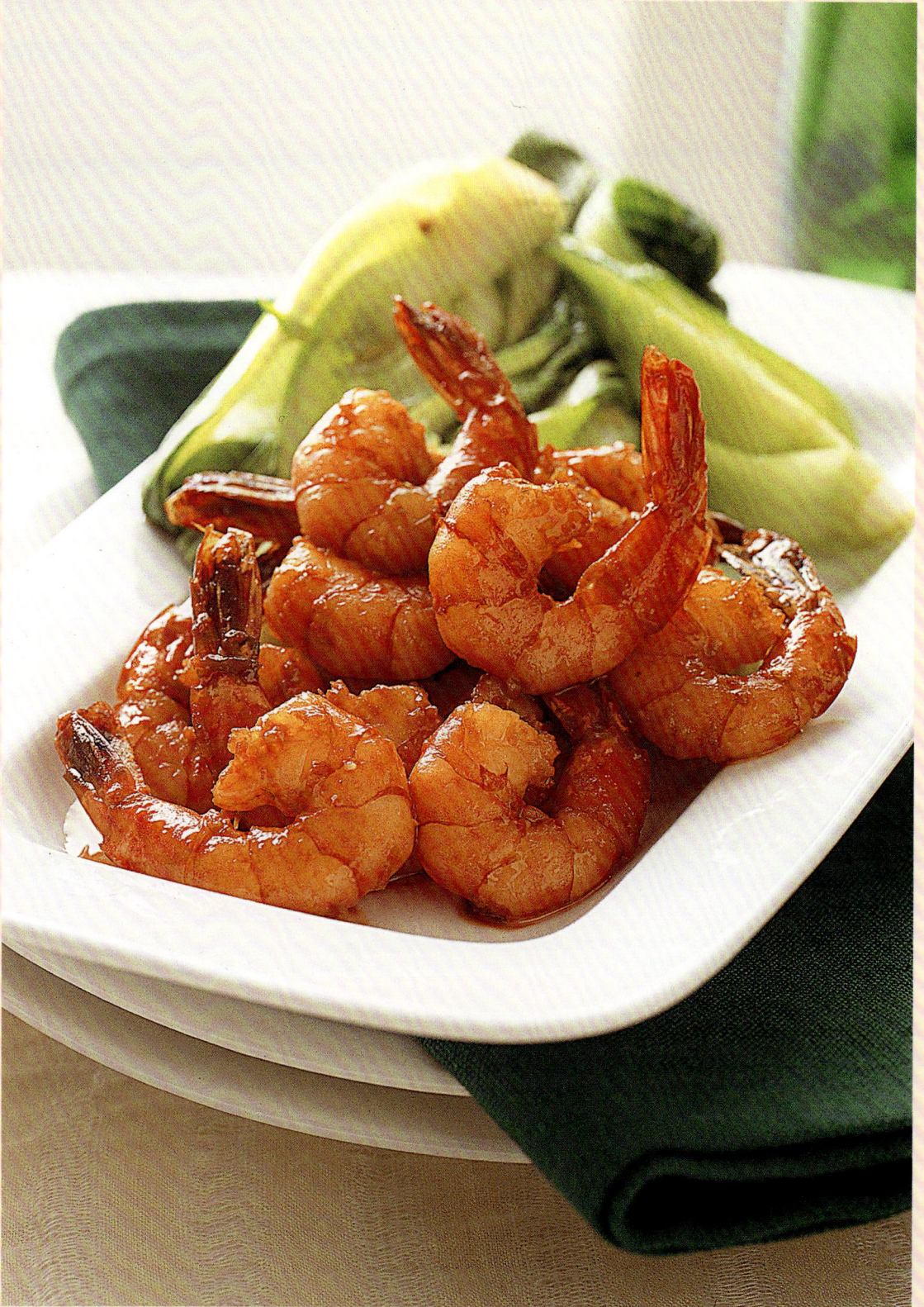

Sesame Prawns
with Pak Choi

Zinc is a key player when it comes to PCOS-supportive minerals. Not only does zinc help to regulate androgens, but it also plays a role in modulating inflammation. Prawns and other shellfish are a great source of zinc, and this sesame prawn with pak choi recipe is a great way to increase your zinc intake in just 10 minutes.

SERVES **4**

600 g (1 lb 3 oz) large frozen peeled
    prawns, defrosted
1 teaspoon sesame oil
2 tablespoons light soy sauce
1 tablespoon clear honey
1 teaspoon grated fresh root ginger
1 teaspoon crushed garlic
1 tablespoon lemon juice
500 g (1 lb) pak choi
2 tablespoons olive oil
salt and pepper

1   Put the prawns in a glass or ceramic bowl. Add the sesame oil, soy sauce, honey, ginger, garlic and lemon juice. Season to taste with salt and pepper and mix well, then cover and leave to marinate in a cool place for 5–10 minutes.

2   Cut the heads of pak choi in half lengthways, then add to a large saucepan of boiling water and blanch for 40–50 seconds. Drain well, cover and keep warm.

3   Heat the olive oil in a wok or large frying pan. Add the prawns and marinade and stir-fry over a high heat for 2 minutes until thoroughly hot.

4   Divide the pak choi between 4 serving plates, then top with the prawns and any juices from the pan. Serve immediately.

Salmon
with Lime Courgettes

These lime courgettes are zesty and fresh, the perfect addition to salmon, a staple PCOS protein. If you feel best eating lower carb, this will be a recipe you'll love!

SERVES **4**

4 salmon fillet portions, about 200 g
    (7 oz) each
1 tablespoon prepared English mustard
1 teaspoon grated fresh root ginger
1 teaspoon crushed garlic
2 teaspoons clear honey
1 tablespoon light soy sauce or tamari
salt and pepper

LIME COURGETTES

2 tablespoons olive oil
500 g (1 lb) courgettes, thinly sliced
    lengthways
grated zest and juice of 1 lime
2 tablespoons chopped mint

1 Lay the salmon fillet portions, skin-side down, in a shallow flameproof dish, to fit snugly in a single layer. In a small bowl, mix together the mustard, ginger, garlic, honey and soy sauce or tamari, then spoon evenly over the fillets. Season to taste with salt and pepper.

2 Heat the grill on the hottest setting. Cook the salmon fillets under the grill for 10–15 minutes, until lightly charred on top and cooked through.

3 Meanwhile, to prepare the lime courgettes, heat the oil in a large nonstick frying pan, add the courgettes and cook, stirring frequently, for 5–6 minutes, or until lightly browned and tender. Stir in the lime zest and juice and chopped mint. Season to taste with salt and pepper.

4 Serve the salmon hot with the courgettes on the side.

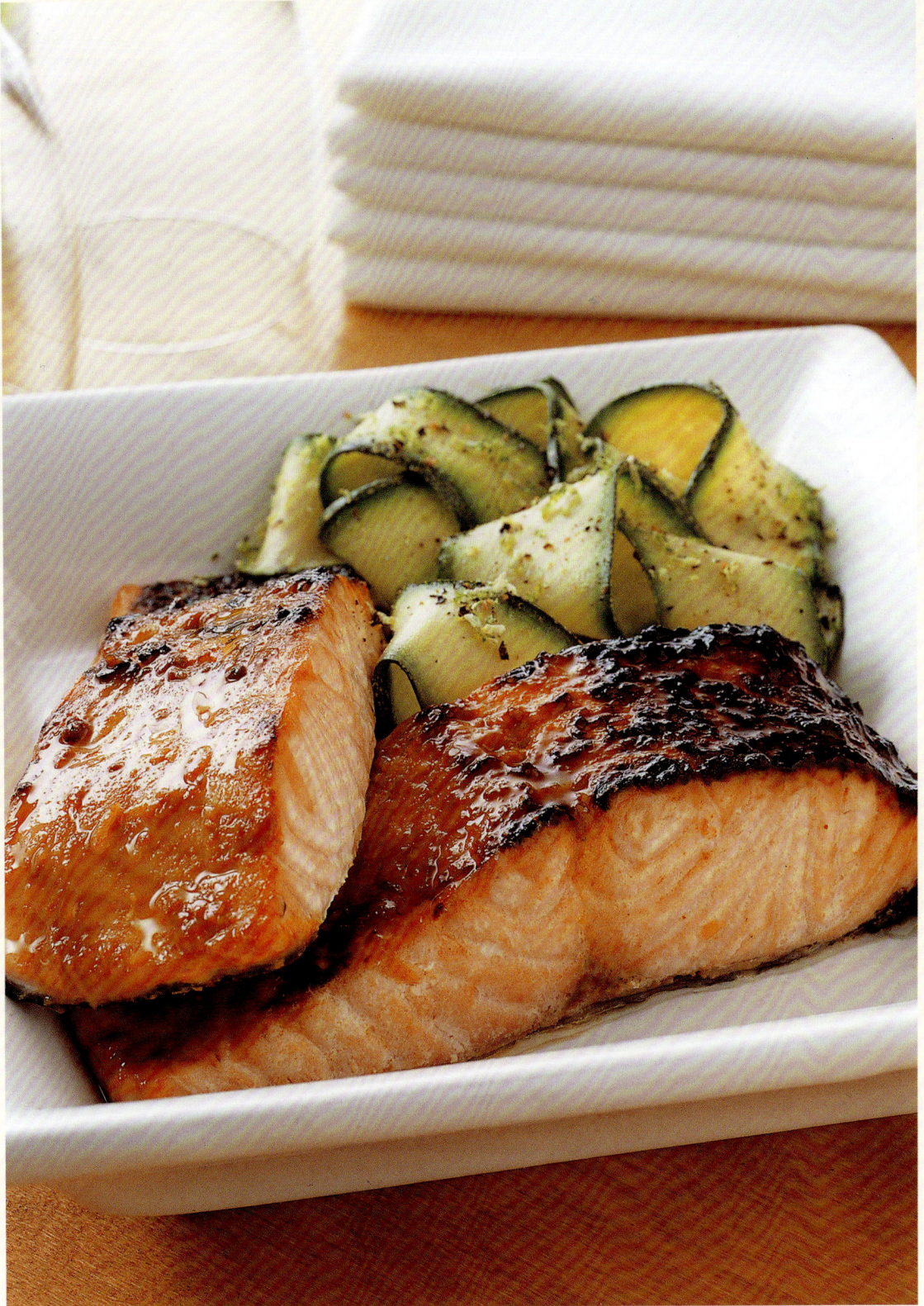

Delicious Dinners

Butternut Squash, Tofu & Pea Curry

Opting for a variety of colourful veggies not only provides your gut with the fibre it needs to maintain a healthy microbiome, but it also means you reap the antioxidant benefits. Antioxidants from plants help to reduce oxidative stress, which can occur in PCOS, impacting ovulation and cardiovascular health. A curry is a great way to cram in colourful plants with ease.

SERVES **4**

1 tablespoon olive oil

1 tablespoon Thai red curry paste

500 g (1 lb) peeled and deseeded butternut
    squash, cubed

450 ml (¾ pint) vegetable stock

400 g (13 oz) can coconut milk

6 makrut lime leaves, bruised, plus
    extra shredded leaves to garnish

200 g (7 oz) frozen peas

300 g (10 oz) firm tofu, diced

2 tablespoons light soy sauce

juice of 1 lime

TO GARNISH
fresh coriander sprigs
finely chopped red chilli

1   Heat the oil in a wok or deep frying pan, add the curry paste and stir-fry over a low heat for 1 minute. Add the squash, stir-fry briefly and then add the stock, coconut milk and the bruised lime leaves. Bring to the boil, then cover, reduce the heat and simmer gently for 15 minutes until the squash is cooked.

2   Stir in the peas, tofu, soy sauce and lime juice and simmer for a further 5 minutes until the peas are cooked.

3   Spoon into serving bowls and garnish with the shredded lime leaves, coriander sprigs and chopped red chilli.

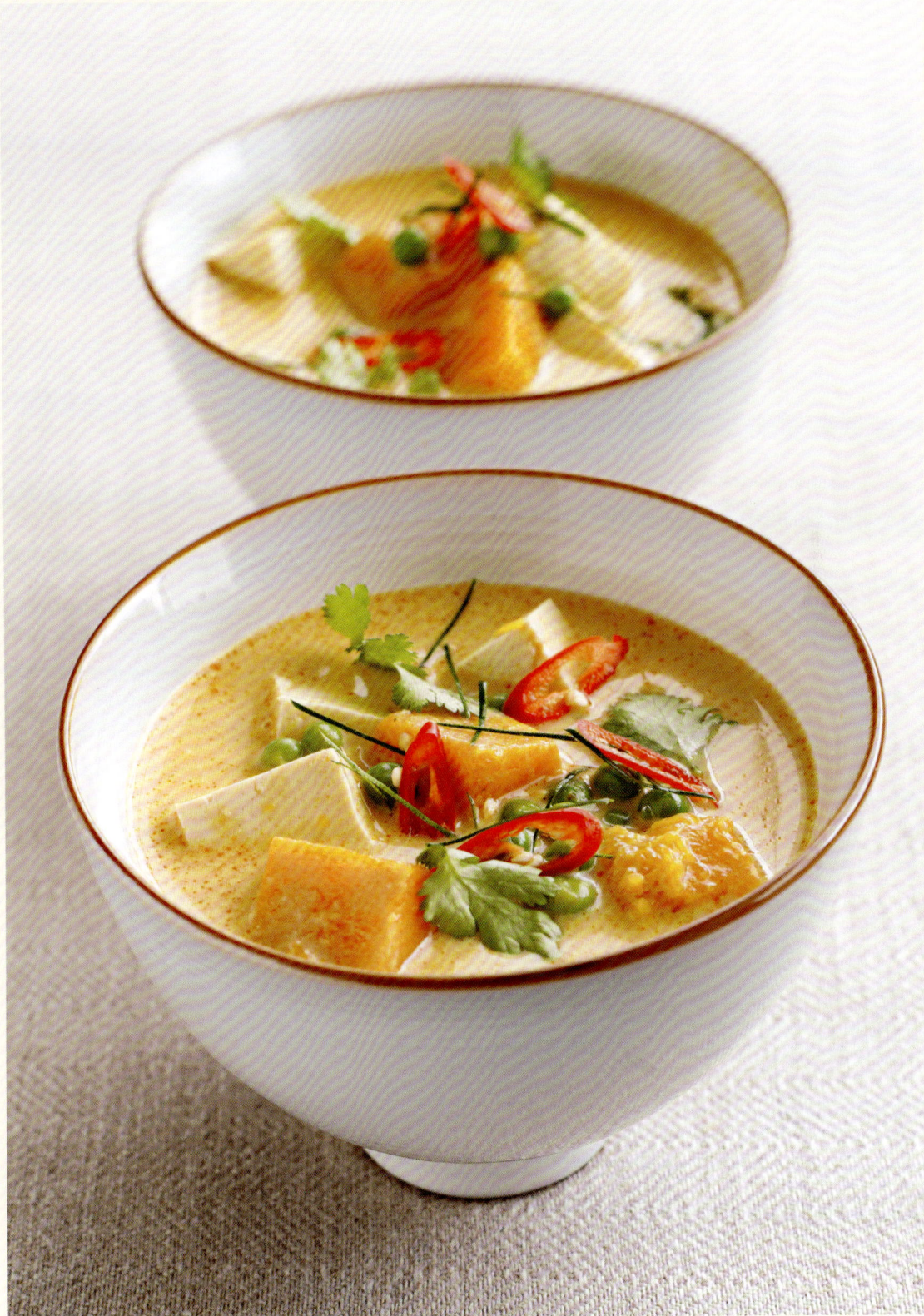

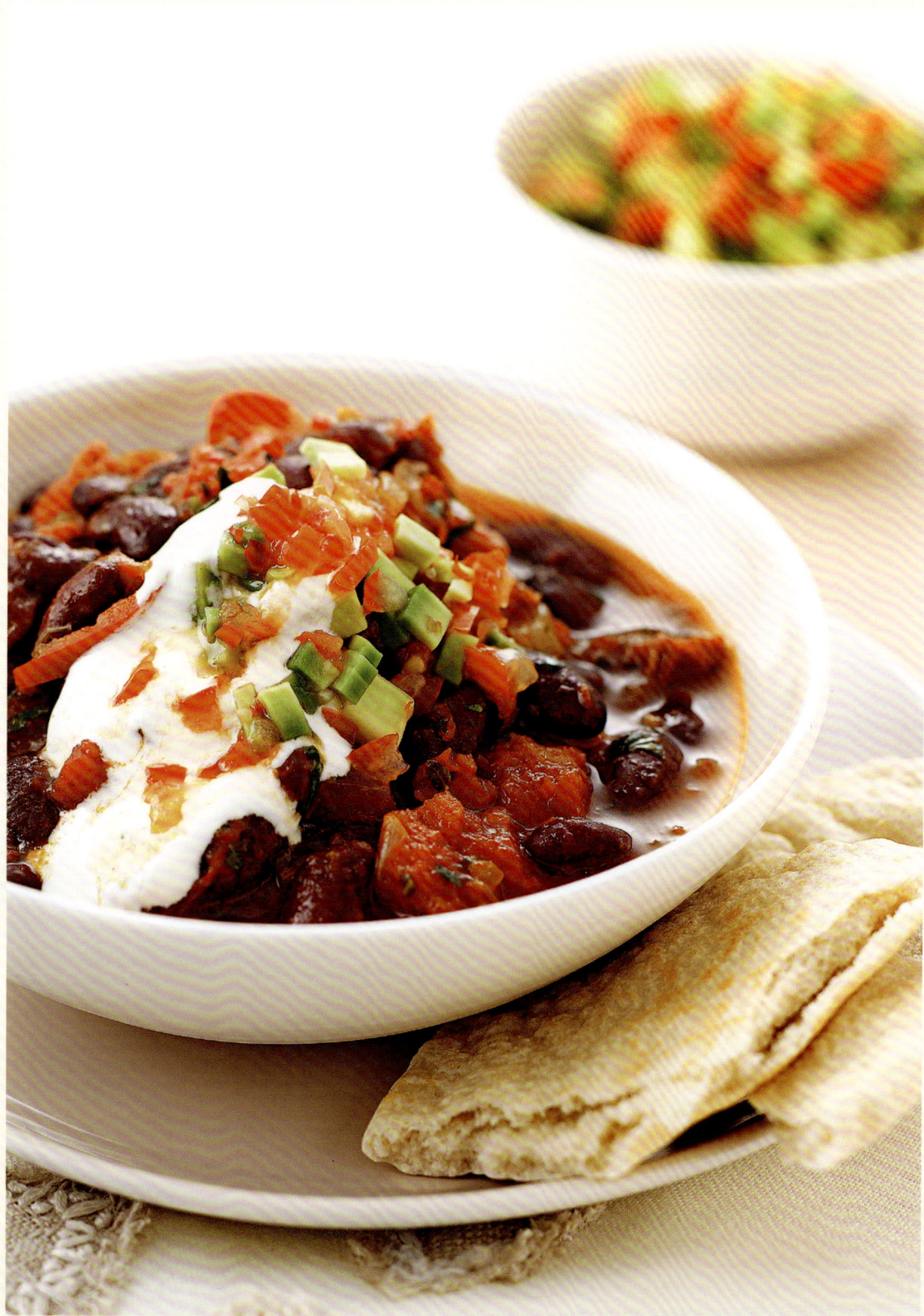

Bean Chilli
with Avocado Salsa

A veggie chilli is a great recipe to have in your repertoire, and it makes for a great go-to for the day before your food shop, when you're utilizing what you have in your store cupboard. Beans are packed with fibre, helping to keep blood sugar levels stable, and contain a variety of different PCOS-friendly vitamins and minerals.

SERVES 4-6

3 tablespoons olive oil

2 teaspoons cumin seeds, crushed

1 teaspoon dried oregano

1 red onion, chopped

1 celery stick, chopped

1 red chilli, deseeded and sliced

2 x 400 g (13 oz) cans chopped tomatoes

50 g (2 oz) sun-dried tomatoes, thinly sliced

300 ml (½ pint) vegetable stock

2 x 400 g (13 oz) cans red kidney beans, drained

handful of coriander, chopped

100 g (3½ oz) natural yogurt

salt and pepper

toasted pitta or flatbreads, to serve

SALSA

1 small avocado

2 tomatoes

2 tablespoons sweet chilli sauce

2 teaspoons lime juice

1 Heat the oil in a large saucepan over a medium-low heat, add the cumin seeds, oregano, onion, celery and chilli and cook gently, stirring frequently, for about 6–8 minutes, or until the vegetables are beginning to colour.

2 Add the canned tomatoes, sun-dried tomatoes, stock, beans and coriander and bring to the boil, then reduce the heat and simmer for about 20 minutes, or until the juices are thickened and pulpy.

3 Make the salsa. Peel, stone and finely dice the avocado and put it in a small bowl. Halve the tomatoes, scoop out the seeds and finely dice the flesh. Add to the bowl along with the chilli sauce and lime juice. Mix well.

4 Season the bean mixture with salt and pepper and spoon into bowls. Top with spoonfuls of natural yogurt and the avocado salsa. Serve with toasted pitta or flatbreads.

Chickpea & Lentil Stew

One easy way to elevate the nutrition of a meal is to get creative with spices. This chickpea and lentil stew incorporates a handful of different anti-inflammatory spices, all deserving of their place in a PCOS-friendly diet. For example, cinnamon can help to regulate blood glucose levels, while the curcumin found in turmeric helps to lower insulin and is a potent antioxidant.

SERVES **4**

200 g (7 oz) dried chickpeas

2 tablespoons olive oil

3 garlic cloves, thinly sliced

1 onion, thinly sliced

1 celery stick, finely diced

2 small carrots, peeled and finely diced

1 teaspoon ground cumin

½ teaspoon ground turmeric

½ teaspoon paprika

½ teaspoon ground ginger

¼ teaspoon ground cinnamon

pinch of saffron threads

125 g (4 oz) green lentils, rinsed

2 tablespoons tomato purée

750 ml (1¼ pints) lamb or vegetable stock

salt and pepper

3–4 tablespoons chopped parsley, to garnish

harissa paste, to serve (optional)

1 Put the chickpeas in a bowl, add cold water to cover by 10 cm (4 inches) and leave to soak overnight.

2 Drain the chickpeas, rinse under running cold water and drain again. Place the chickpeas in a saucepan of cold water and bring to the boil. Boil rapidly for 10 minutes, then reduce the heat and simmer gently, partially covered, for about 1 hour or until tender, adding more water as necessary. Drain well.

3 Meanwhile, heat the oil in a large saucepan over a medium-low heat, add the garlic, onion, celery and carrots and cook for 15 minutes, or until softened, stirring frequently. Add the spices and cook for 1–2 minutes, then increase the heat and add the chickpeas, lentils and tomato purée. Pour in the stock and bring to the boil, then reduce the heat and simmer gently for 40–45 minutes.

4 Spoon the pulses and vegetables into serving bowls and carefully pour the liquid around the side. Sprinkle with parsley and serve with harissa, to taste.

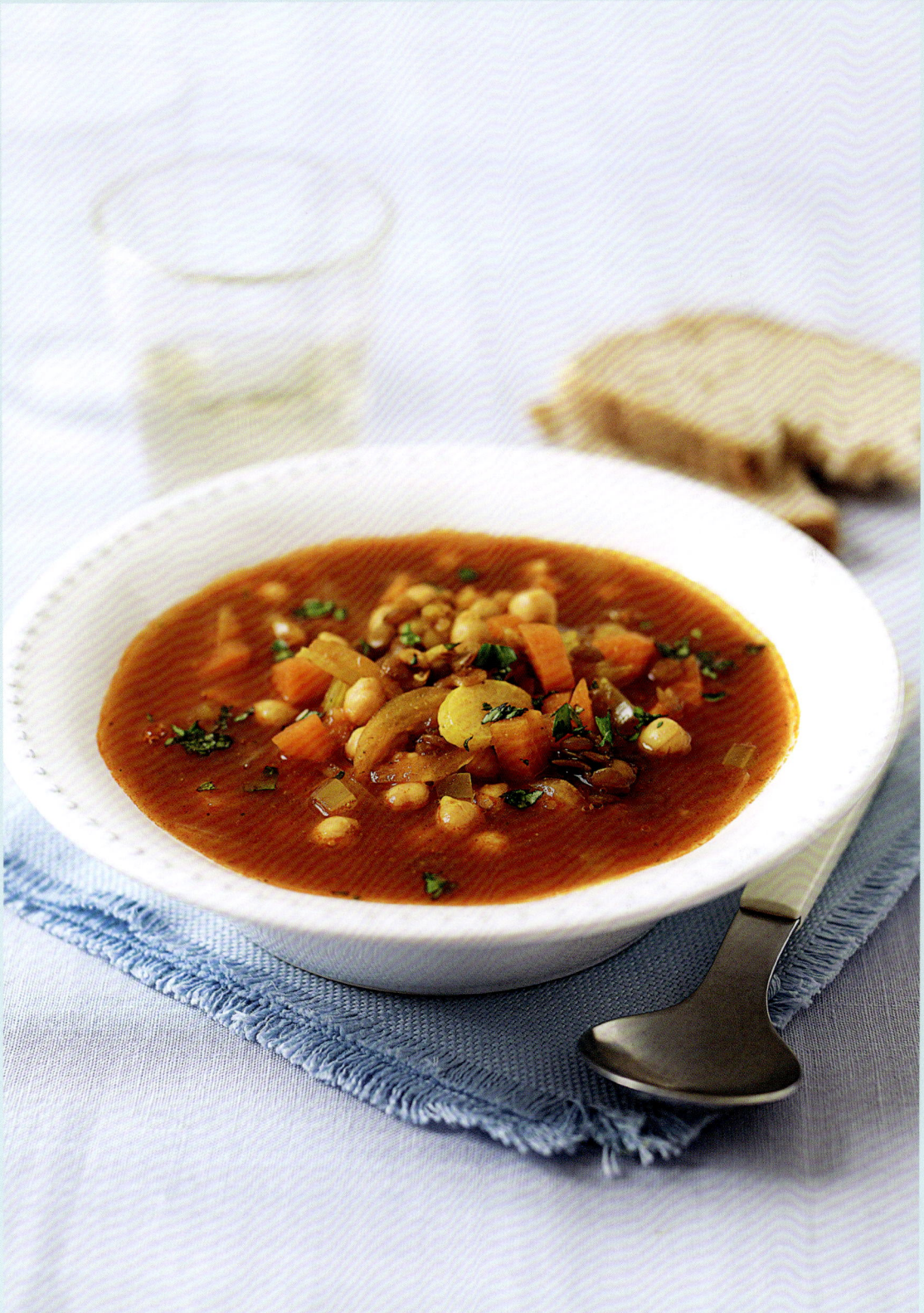

Cajun-spiced Turkey Meatballs

In this delicious dinner, the protein and complex carbohydrate pairing, from the turkey and the sweet potato, helps keep blood sugar levels stable, which in turn aids hormone balance.

SERVES 4

1 kg (2 lb) sweet potatoes, cut into
    thin wedges
4 tablespoons olive oil
1 small red onion, sliced
1 red pepper, deseeded and sliced
2 garlic cloves
4 teaspoons Cajun-style spice blend
680 g (1 lb 6 oz) jar passata
salt and pepper
natural yogurt, to serve (optional)

MEATBALLS

500 g (1 lb) minced turkey
2 teaspoons Cajun-style spice blend
2 spring onions, finely chopped
50 g (2 oz) almond flour
2 tablespoons chopped coriander

1   Place the sweet potatoes in a roasting tin with half of the oil and season. Toss well, then roast in a preheated oven, 220 °C (425 °F), Gas Mark 7, for 20–25 minutes, until golden and tender.

2   Meanwhile, combine all the meatball ingredients in a bowl, adding some salt and pepper. Roll into 20–24 balls. Heat the remaining oil in a large pan and cook the meatballs over a medium-high heat for 3–4 minutes, shaking the pan occasionally, until browned. Transfer to a plate and set aside.

3   Return the oily pan to the heat and cook the onion, pepper and garlic for 7–8 minutes until softened and lightly coloured. Add the spice mix and stir over a medium heat for 1 minute. Pour in the passata, add a pinch of salt and pepper and simmer for 5–6 minutes to thicken the sauce slightly.

4   Add the meatballs to the sauce and simmer for a further 6–7 minutes until cooked and the sauce has thickened. Serve with the sweet potato wedges and a dollop of natural yogurt, if desired.

tip | No turkey mince on hand? Chicken mince works just as well.

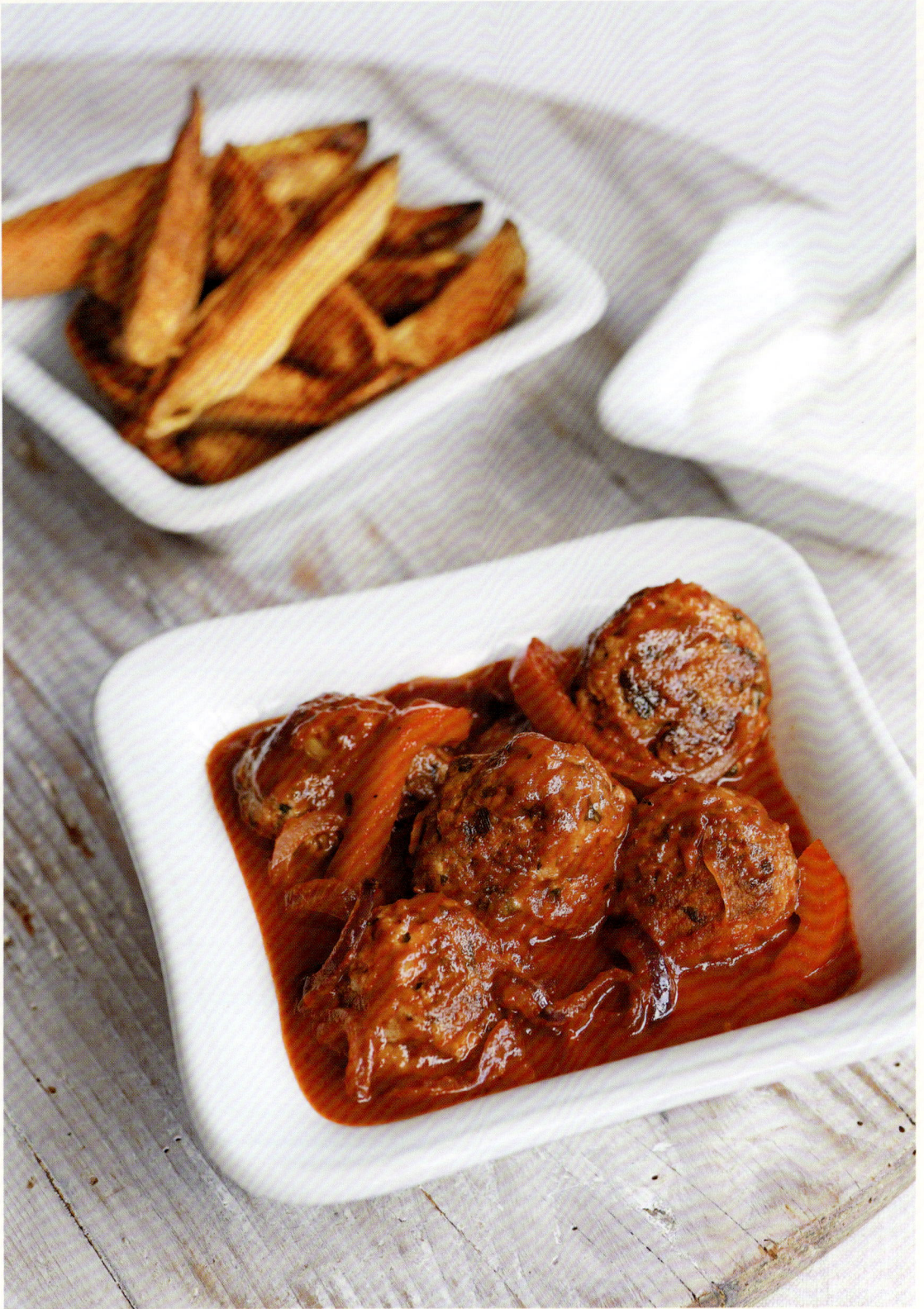

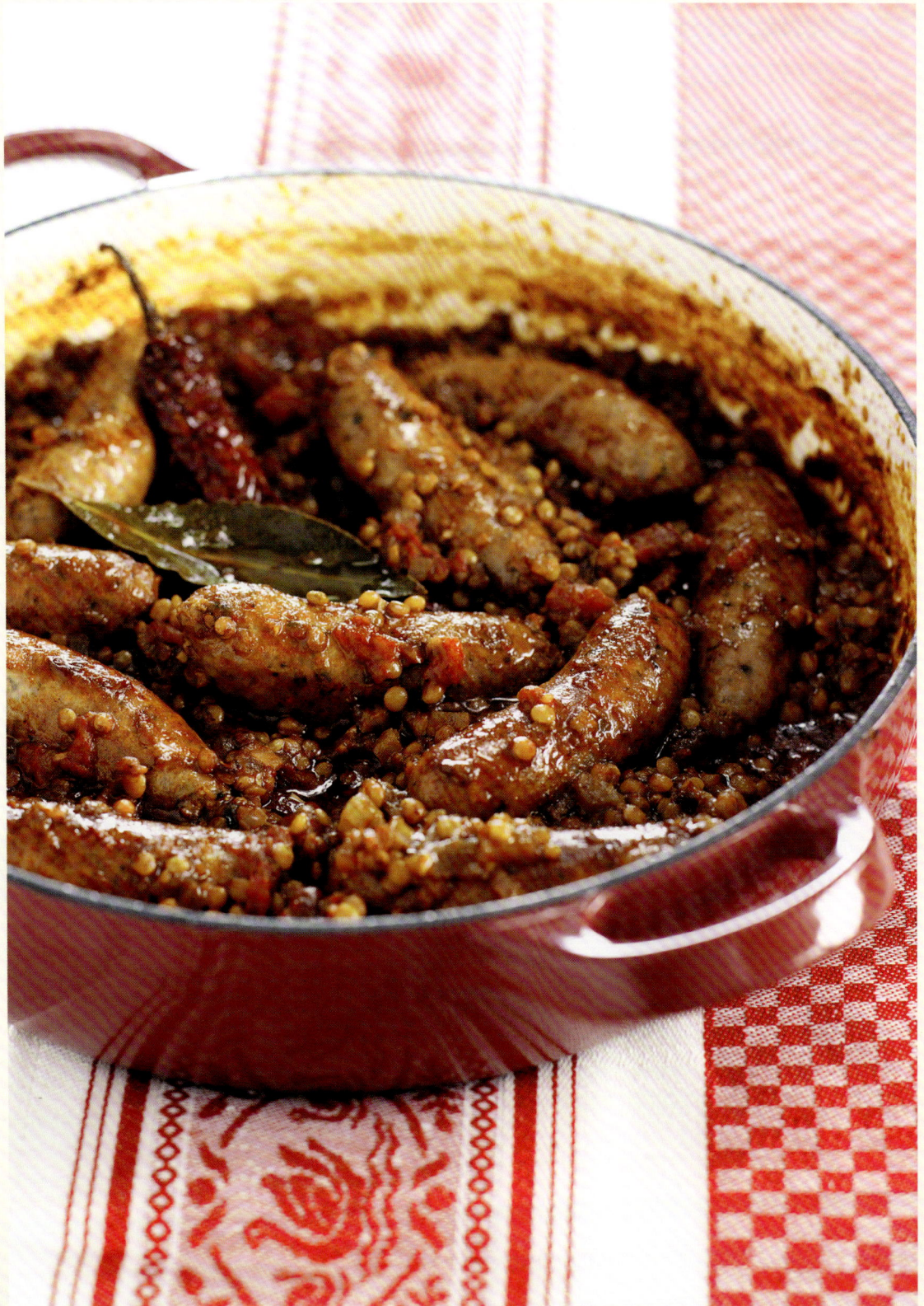

Sausages & Lentils
in Tomato Sauce

Fan of sausages? Consider incorporating chicken sausages into your dinners. They are a great PCOS-friendly staple to have on hand, due to their lean protein content. This high-protein, high-fibre sausage and lentil dish is a nutritious choice if you're looking for something hearty and satiating at the end of a long day.

SERVES 4

3 tablespoons olive oil

8 chicken sausages

1 onion, roughly chopped

1 celery stick, roughly chopped

3 garlic cloves, crushed

200 ml (7 fl oz) full-bodied red wine

400 g (13 oz) can chopped tomatoes

1.2 litres (2 pints) chicken stock

1 bay leaf

1 dried red chilli

125 g (4 oz) green lentils

salt and pepper

TO SERVE

extra virgin olive oil, for drizzling

crusty bread

1   Heat the olive oil in a large, heavy-based saucepan in which the sausages fit in a single layer. Add the sausages and cook over a medium heat for 10–12 minutes until golden brown all over. Remove and set aside.

2   Add the onion and celery to the pan and cook over a low heat for 8–10 minutes until softened. Stir in the garlic and cook for a further 2 minutes.

3   Increase the heat to high, pour in the wine and boil vigorously for 2 minutes, scraping any sediment from the base of the pan. Stir in the tomatoes, stock, bay leaf and chilli and bring to the boil. Add the lentils and return the sausages to the pan. Simmer gently for 40 minutes, or until the sausages and lentils are cooked through. Season with salt and pepper.

4   Serve with a drizzle of extra virgin olive oil, alongside some crusty bread.

Lamb & Spinach Curry

Lamb is incredibly nutrient-dense, rich in zinc for healthy androgen activity and a number of B vitamins, which aid in balanced mood, energy levels and sleep. When you cook lamb low and slow, it falls apart with ease and almost melts in your mouth, making it a decadent and delicious way of getting your protein in.

SERVES **4**

4 tablespoons olive oil

600 g (1 lb 4 oz) boneless shoulder of
    lamb, cut into bite-sized pieces

1 onion, finely chopped

3 garlic cloves, crushed

1 teaspoon ground ginger

2 teaspoons ground turmeric

large pinch of grated nutmeg

4 tablespoons sultanas

1 teaspoon ground cinnamon

1 teaspoon paprika

400 g (13 oz) canned chopped tomatoes

300 ml (½ pint) lamb stock

400 g (13 oz) baby leaf spinach

salt and pepper

whisked natural yogurt, to serve (optional)

1   Heat half of the oil in a large, heavy-based saucepan and brown the lamb, in batches, for 3–4 minutes. Remove with a slotted spoon and set aside.

2   Heat the remaining oil in the pan and add the onion, garlic, ginger, turmeric, nutmeg, sultanas, cinnamon and paprika. Stir-fry for 1–2 minutes, then add the lamb. Stir-fry for 2–3 minutes and then add the tomatoes and stock. Season well and bring to the boil, then reduce the heat, cover tightly and simmer very gently (using a heat diffuser, if possible) for 1½ hours.

3   Add the spinach in batches until it is all wilted, cover and cook for a further 10–12 minutes, stirring occasionally. Remove from the heat and serve drizzled with whisked yogurt, if liked.

tip | Beef also works very well in this dish.

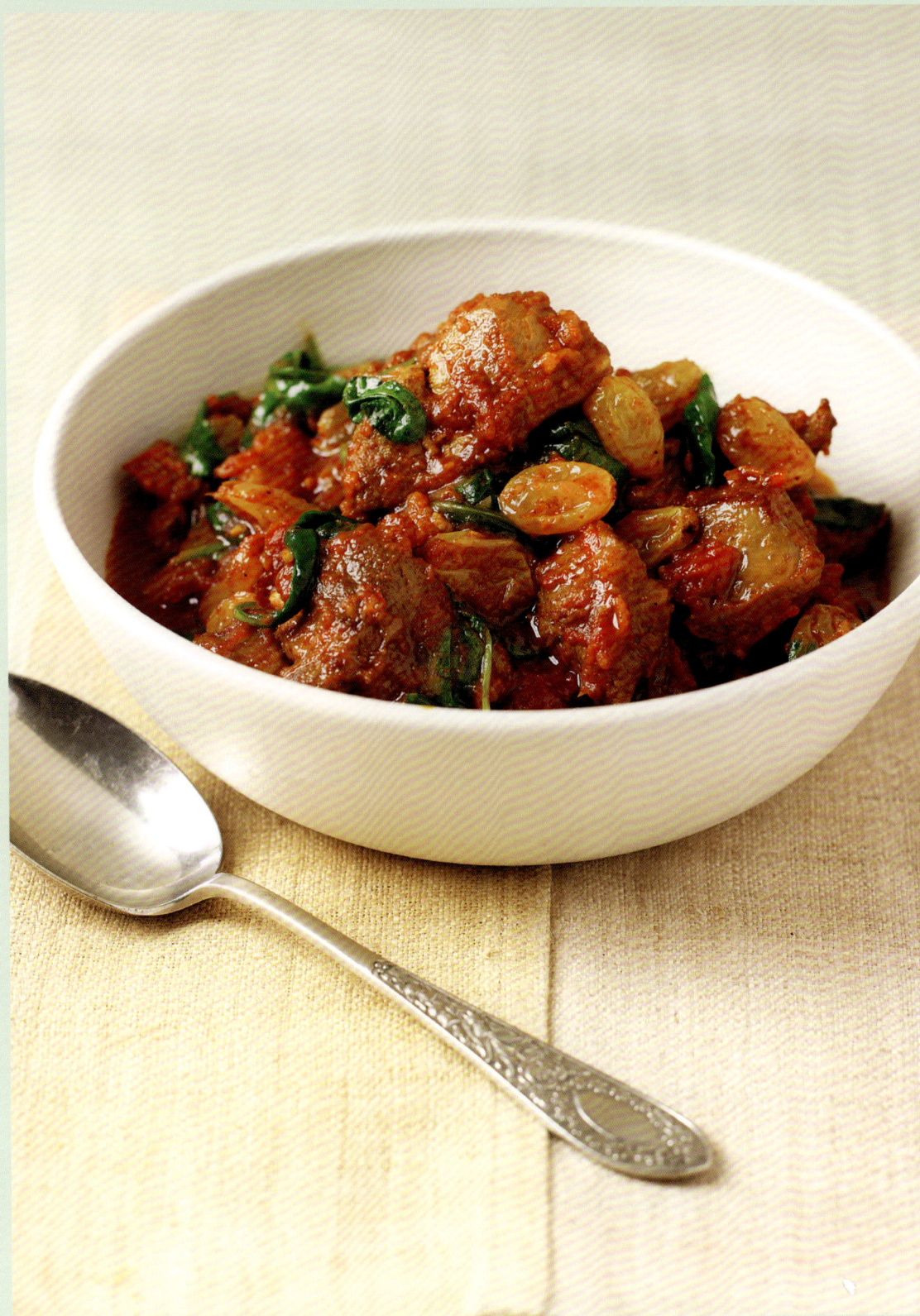

Turkey Burgers
with Sweet Potato Wedges

When you receive a PCOS diagnosis and are told that you may need to be a little more cautious with your diet, it might feel as though you've been cut off from all your favourite foods. Making small tweaks and healthier versions of the meals that you love can help to reduce any feelings of restriction and help healthy eating feel like more of a longer-term, sustainable lifestyle change rather than a quick-fix diet.

SERVES **4**

750 g (1½ lb) sweet potatoes, washed
    but unpeeled and cut into wedges
2 tablespoons olive oil
500 g (1 lb) turkey mince
½ red pepper, cored, deseeded
    and chopped
325 g (11 oz) can sweetcorn, rinsed
    and drained
1 onion, chopped
1 egg, beaten
6 wholemeal bread rolls
salt and pepper
salad leaves and tomato slices,
    to serve

1 Toss the potato wedges in 1 tablespoon of the oil, season to taste and bake in a preheated oven, 200°C (400°F), Gas Mark 6, for 30 minutes, turning after 15 minutes.

2 Meanwhile, in a large bowl mix together the mince with the red pepper, sweetcorn and onion. Season to taste and add the egg. Shape the mixture into 6 burgers and refrigerate until ready to cook.

3 Heat the remaining oil in a shallow frying pan over a medium heat. Add the burgers, 3 at a time, and cook for 2 minutes on each side until brown. Transfer to a baking sheet and finish cooking in the oven, below the potato wedges, for 15 minutes, or until cooked through.

4 Cut the rolls in half and toast them, cut-sides down, in the hot pan. Put a few salad leaves and tomato slices in each roll, add a burger and serve them with the sweet potato wedges.

tip | Add a couple of slices of avocado on top of your burger for some healthy fats!

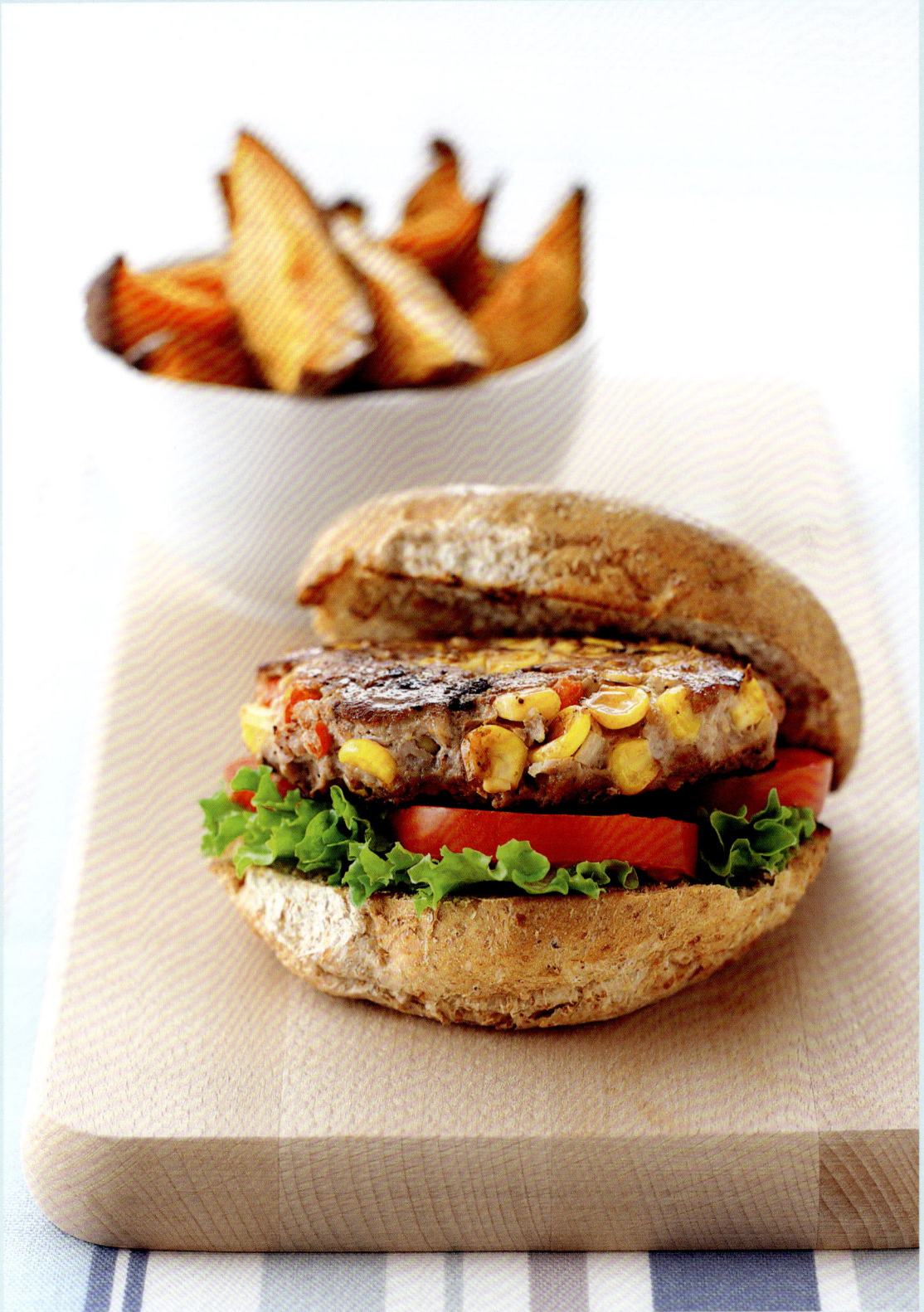

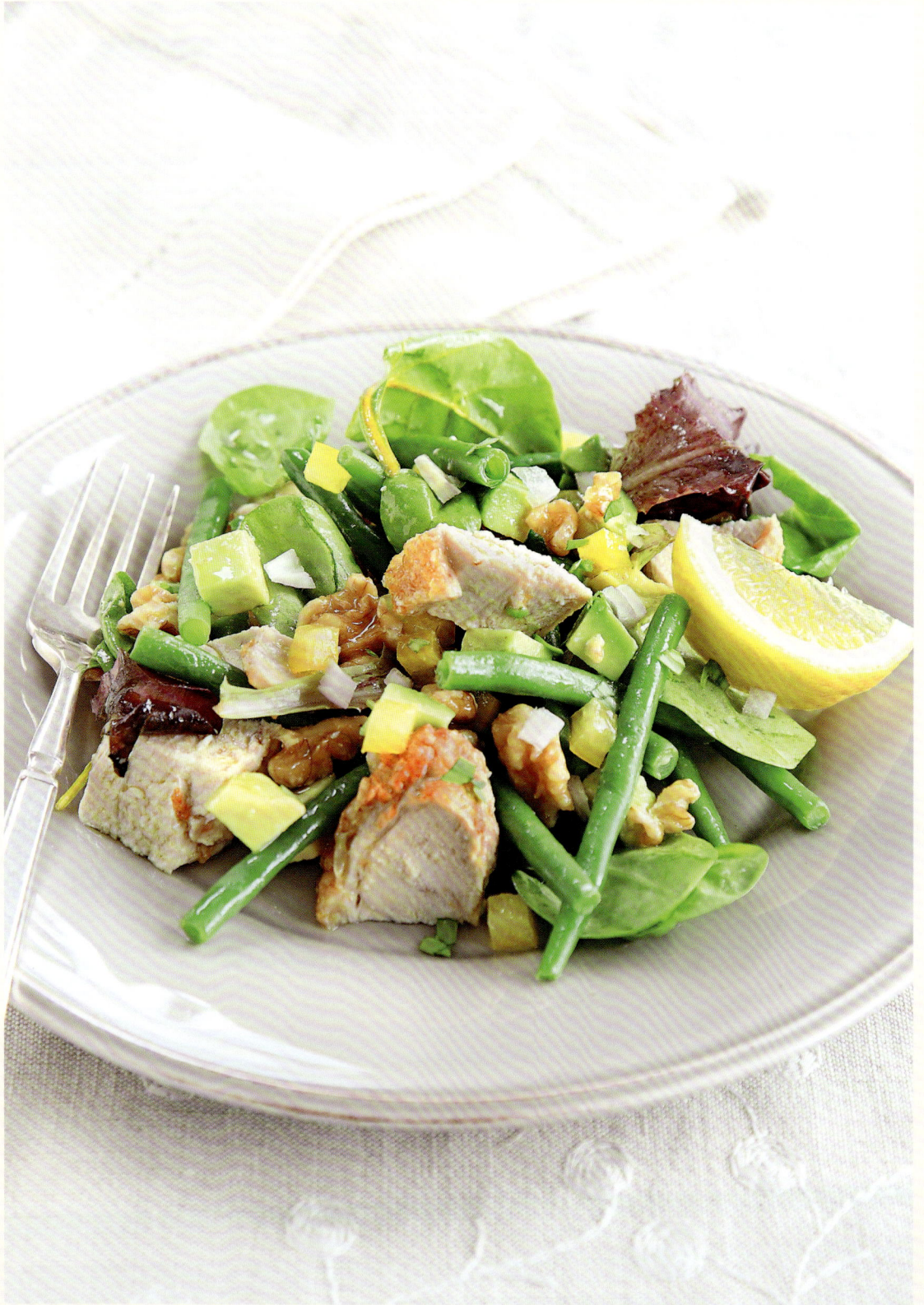

Chicken
with Beans, Walnuts & Tarragon

If salads leave you feeling hungry shortly after putting down your fork, upping the protein and fibre content may just be the thing to increase satiety. Including a complete, lean protein source, such as chicken, alongside a high-fibre legume boosts the nutritional density and helps to keep you fuller for longer. Finishing a salad with healthy fats, like alpha-linolenic acid (ALA)-rich walnuts, further stabilizes blood sugar levels and gives your brain a boost.

SERVES **4**

200 g (7 oz) fine green beans, trimmed

1 firm, ripe avocado, stoned and peeled

1 tablespoon lemon juice

175 g (7 oz) mesclun or mixed leaf salad

300 g (10 oz) cooked whole chicken
    breasts, roughly chopped

1 yellow pepper, finely chopped

50 g (2 oz) walnut pieces

1 shallot, finely chopped (optional)

2 teaspoons chopped tarragon

4 teaspoons walnut oil

salt and pepper

lemon wedges, to serve

1   Bring a small saucepan of lightly salted water to the boil. When the water is boiling add the beans and cook for 3–4 minutes until just tender, then drain and cool under running cold water.

2   Meanwhile, dice the flesh of the avocado and toss in the lemon juice to prevent it from turning brown.

3   Place the mesclun or mixed leaf salad in a large bowl. Add the chicken, pepper, walnuts, beans and avocado, then gently toss until well combined.

4   Heap the salad onto serving plates and sprinkle over the shallot, if using, and tarragon. Season with a little salt and plenty of pepper, then drizzle over the walnut oil. Serve immediately with lemon wedges, perhaps with some nutty granary bread on the side.

Chicken, Okra & Red Lentil Dhal

There's nothing quite as comforting as a bowl of dhal after a long day. Lentils provide a hearty, high-fibre base for this dish and come with a number of PCOS-friendly micronutrients including folate and potassium, supporting energy levels and heart health. Adding a complete protein source, such as chicken, is a great way to keep your blood sugar levels stable while including good amounts of the sleep-promoting amino acid l-tryptophan.

SERVES **4**

2 teaspoons ground cumin

1 teaspoon ground coriander

½ teaspoon cayenne pepper

¼ teaspoon ground turmeric

500 g (1 lb) skinless, boneless chicken thighs, cut into large pieces

2 tablespoons groundnut oil

1 onion, sliced

2 garlic cloves, crushed

25 g (1 oz) fresh root ginger, peeled and finely chopped

750 ml (1¼ pints) water

300 g (10 oz) red lentils, rinsed

200 g (7 oz) okra, trimmed

small handful of coriander leaves, chopped

salt

lime wedges, to serve

1   Mix the cumin, coriander, cayenne and turmeric in a bowl and toss with the chicken pieces.

2   Heat the oil in a large saucepan. Fry the chicken pieces in batches until deeply golden, transferring each batch to a plate. Add the onion to the pan and fry for 5 minutes until golden. Stir in the garlic and ginger and cook for a further 1 minute.

3   Return the chicken to the pan and add the measured water. Bring to the boil, reduce the heat and simmer very gently, covered, for 20 minutes until the chicken is cooked through. Add the lentils and cook for 5 minutes.

4   Stir in the okra, coriander and a little salt and cook for a further 5 minutes until the lentils are tender but not completely pulpy. Serve in shallow bowls with lime wedges.

tip | For a meat-free variation, swap the chicken for tofu.

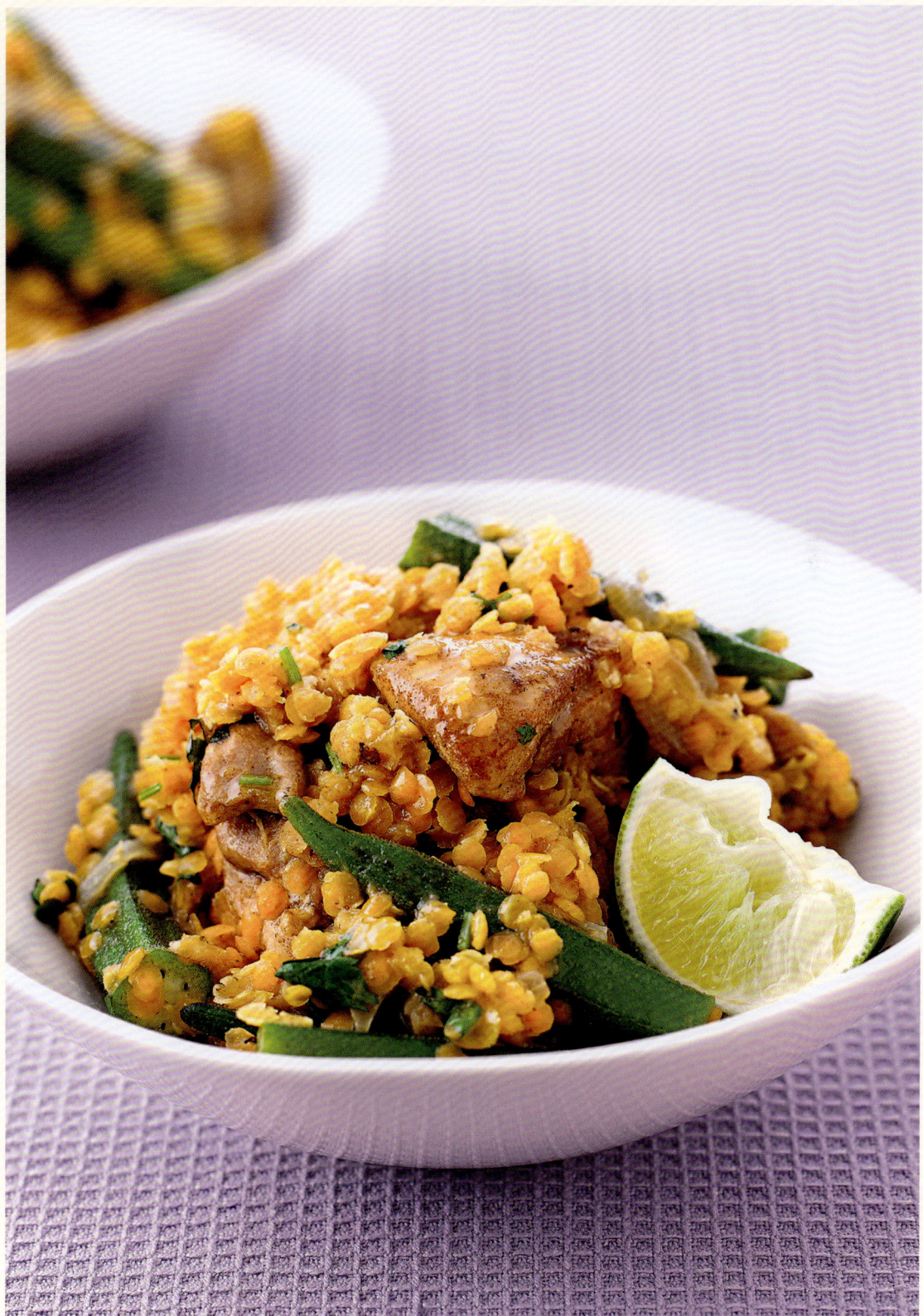

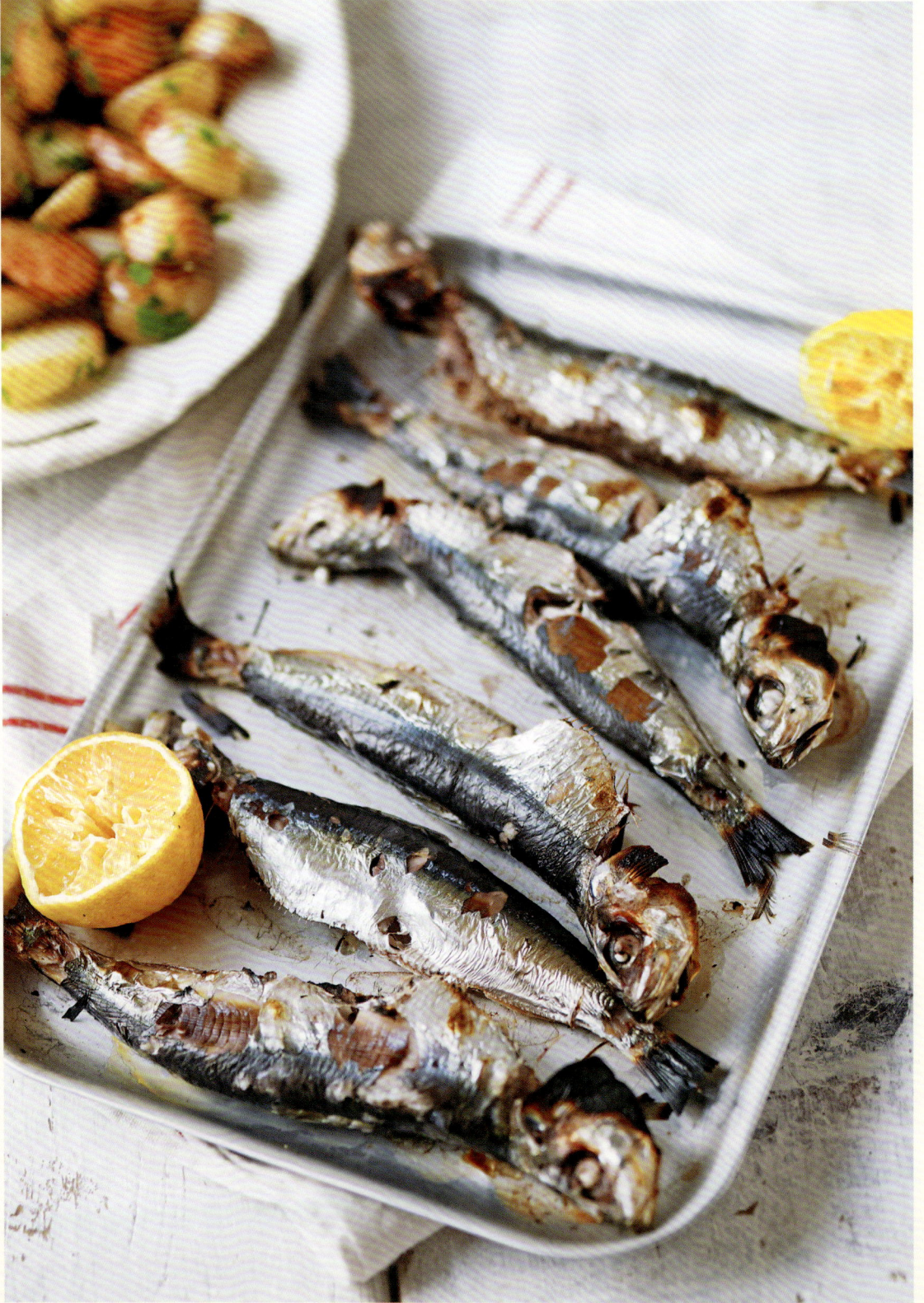

Grilled Sardines
with Pan-fried Potatoes

The Mediterranean diet is the most studied diet and is used as a therapeutic tool for many different conditions. PCOS is no exception, and opting for a Mediterranean-style diet may help to reduce inflammation that paves the way for insulin resistance and hyperandrogenemia. This recipe is the perfect example of how you can utilize Mediterranean staples, such as oily fish, citrus, olive oil and whole carbohydrates.

SERVES 4

625 g (1¼ lb) new potatoes, thickly sliced
1 tablespoon olive oil
12 sardines, cleaned and gutted
grated zest and juice of 1 lemon
2 tablespoons chopped parsley

1 Cook the potatoes in boiling water for 12–15 minutes until tender.

2 Heat the oil in a frying pan over a medium heat, add the potatoes and cook for 6–8 minutes, turning regularly until golden.

3 Meanwhile, place the sardines on a grill tray and squeeze over the lemon juice. Cook the sardines under a preheated hot grill for 2–3 minutes on each side.

4 Toss the lemon zest and chopped parsley into the potatoes and serve with the grilled sardines.

Salmon & Puy Lentils
with Parsley

Mixing up your carbohydrates is a great way to increase overall nutrient density in your meals. Including a variety of different types of plants also feeds your gut microbes with a diverse range of fibre and polyphenols. Instead of rice with your salmon, try Puy lentils, dressed up with herbs and citrus for a fresh flavour.

SERVES **4**

200 g (7 oz) Puy lentils

1 bay leaf

200 g (7 oz) fine green beans, chopped

25 g (1 oz) flat leaf parsley, chopped

2 tablespoons Dijon mustard

2 tablespoons capers, rinsed and chopped

2 tablespoons olive oil

2 lemons, finely sliced

about 500 g (1 lb) salmon fillets

1 fennel bulb, finely sliced

salt and pepper

dill sprigs, to garnish

1 Put the lentils into a saucepan with the bay leaf and enough cold water to cover (do not add salt). Bring to the boil, reduce to a simmer and cook for 30 minutes, or until tender. Season to taste, add the beans and simmer for 1 minute. Drain the lentils and stir in the parsley, mustard, capers and oil. Discard the bay leaf.

2 Meanwhile, arrange the lemon slices on a foil-lined grill pan and put the salmon and fennel slices on top. Season the salmon and fennel and cook under a preheated hot grill for about 10 minutes, or until the salmon is cooked through.

3 Serve the fennel and lemon slices and lentils with the salmon on top, garnished with dill sprigs.

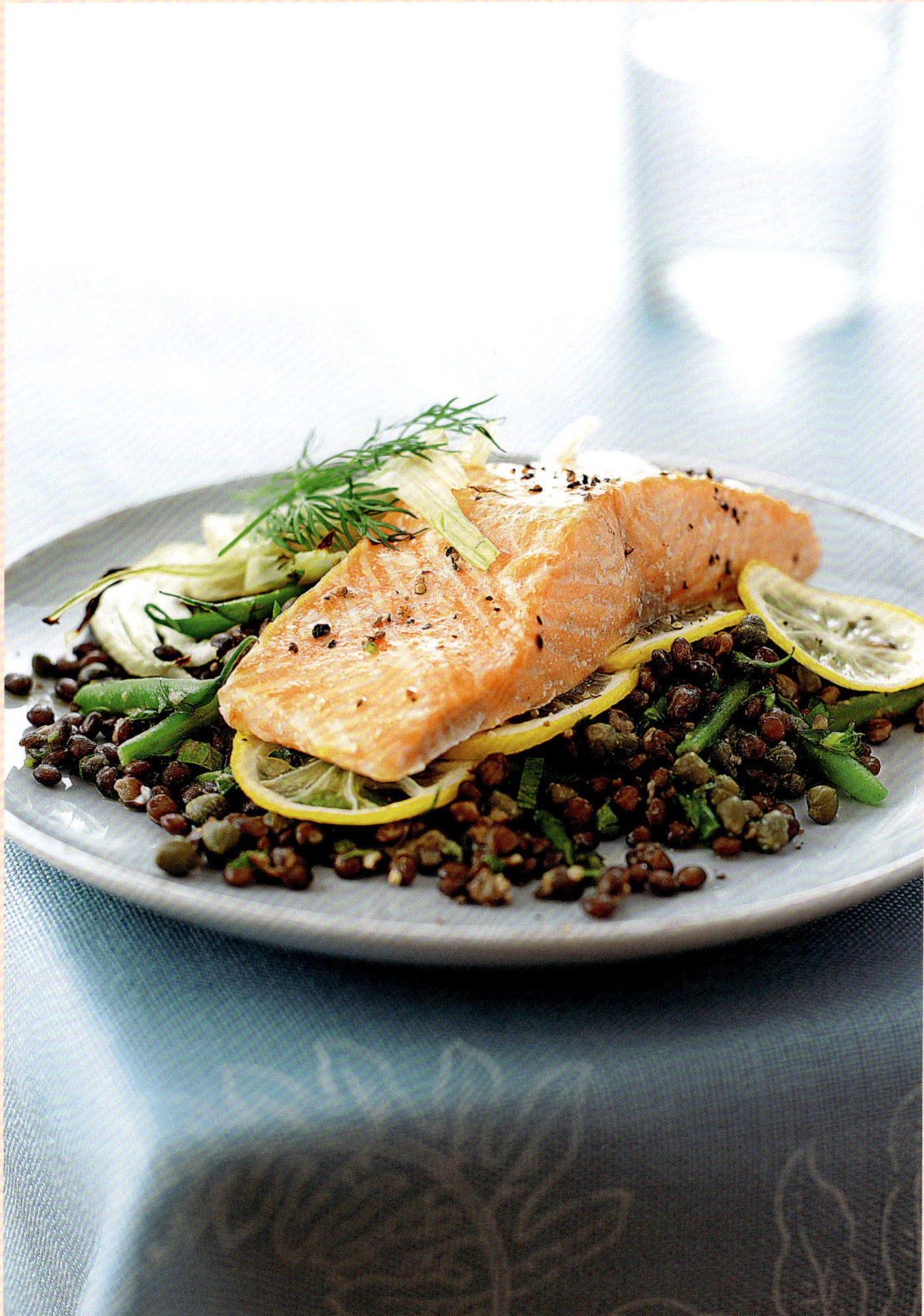

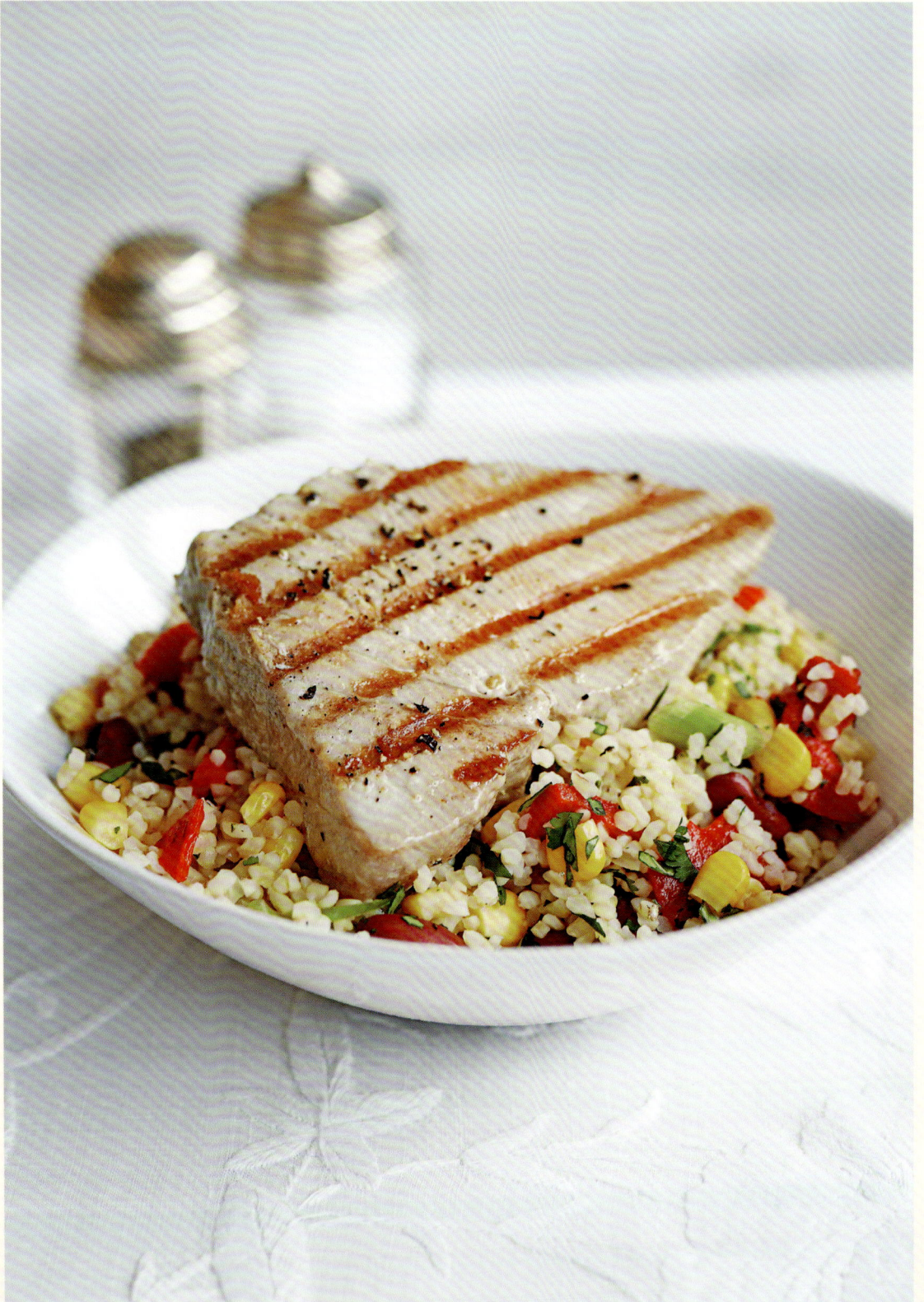

Tuna & Bulgur Wheat Bowl

Increasing the diversity of colourful plants in your diet is a great way to automatically increase your intake of antioxidants, vitamins and minerals. This tuna and bulgur wheat bowl is as diverse as it gets, containing vegetables, a source of wholegrains and legumes, and fresh herbs. Add tuna for the bioavailable protein, selenium and vitamin B6 and you have a well-rounded PCOS dinner.

SERVES 4

750 ml (1¼ pints) vegetable stock
300 g (10 oz) bulgur wheat
3 tablespoons olive oil
4 tuna steaks
400 g (13 oz) can kidney beans, drained
125 g (4 oz) drained or defrosted
    sweetcorn
2 spring onions, finely sliced
2 roasted red peppers, drained
    and diced
small bunch of coriander, chopped
2 tablespoons lemon juice
salt and pepper

1 Pour the stock into a pan, bring to the boil and add the bulgur. Cook, uncovered, over a medium heat for 7 minutes. Cover with a tight-fitting lid and set aside for 6–7 minutes until the liquid has been absorbed and the grains are tender.

2 Meanwhile, heat a ridged griddle pan over a medium-high heat. Rub 1 tablespoon of the oil over the tuna steaks and season with salt and pepper. Cook them in the griddle pan for 2–3 minutes on each side until nicely charred and cooked to your liking. Set aside and keep warm.

3 Gently stir the remaining ingredients into the bulgur, then replace the lid for 3–4 minutes. Spoon the warm mixture into bowls and serve topped with the griddled tuna.

Baked Cod
with Tomatoes & Olives

Cod pairs perfectly with tomatoes and olives, transforming this simple, meaty fish into a vibrant Mediterranean dish. Cod is a great source of iodine, which is an essential mineral for optimal thyroid function. Hypothyroidism is more common in women with PCOS, so consider incorporating sufficient amounts of thyroid-healthy nutrients, including iodine, selenium and zinc, in your meals.

SERVES **4**

250 g (8 oz) cherry tomatoes, halved
100 g (3½ oz) pitted black olives
2 tablespoons capers in brine, drained
4 thyme sprigs, plus extra for garnish
4 cod fillets, about 175 g (6 oz) each
2 tablespoons extra virgin olive oil
2 tablespoons balsamic vinegar
salt and black pepper

1 Combine the tomatoes, olives, capers and thyme sprigs in a roasting tin. Nestle the cod fillets in the pan, drizzle over the oil and balsamic vinegar and season to taste with salt and pepper.

2 Bake in a preheated oven, 200°C (400°F), Gas Mark 6, for 15 minutes.

3 Transfer the fish, tomatoes and olives to warmed plates. Spoon the pan juices over the fish. Serve immediately, garnished with extra thyme sprigs, with a mixed green leaf salad.

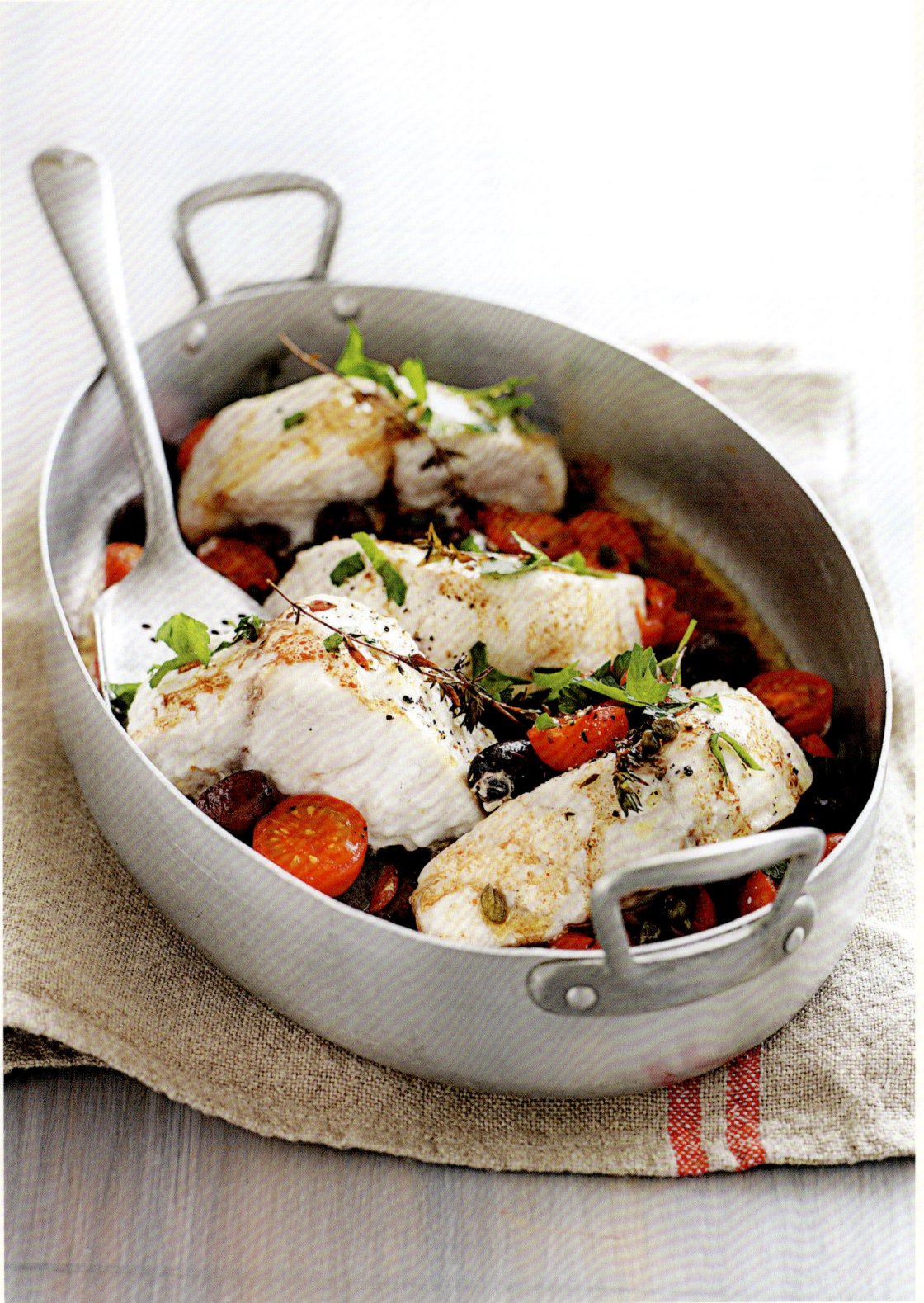

Salmon Fillets
with Sage & Quinoa

Great, healthy recipes don't have to be complicated, and sometimes the tastiest ones call on simple, delicious ingredients to make them great. Salmon is rich in omega-3 fatty acids, while quinoa contains lots of fibre and tops up the protein profile of the meal.

SERVES 4

200 g (7 oz) quinoa

100 g (3½ oz) butter, at room temperature

8 sage leaves, chopped

small bunch of chives

grated zest and juice of 1 lemon

4 salmon fillet steaks,
    about 125 g (4 oz) each

1 tablespoon olive oil

salt and pepper

1   Cook the quinoa in unsalted boiling water for about 15 minutes, or until cooked but firm.

2   Meanwhile, mix the butter with the sage, chives and lemon zest. Add salt and pepper to taste.

3   Rub the salmon steaks with the oil, season with pepper and cook in a preheated hot griddle pan for about 6 minutes, turning carefully once. Remove and set aside to rest.

4   Drain the quinoa, stir in the lemon juice and season to taste. Spoon on to serving plates and top with the salmon, topping each piece with a knob of sage butter.

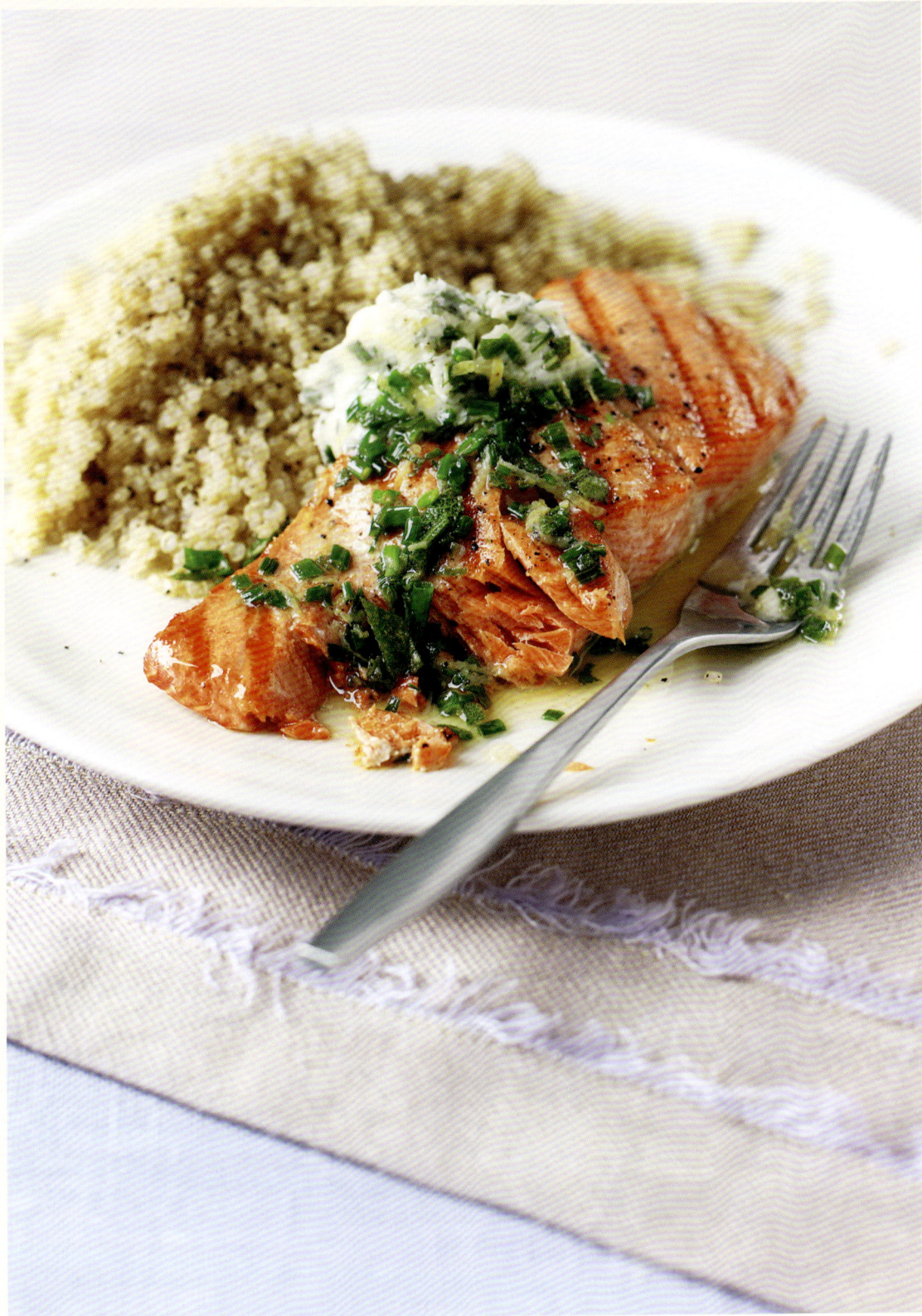

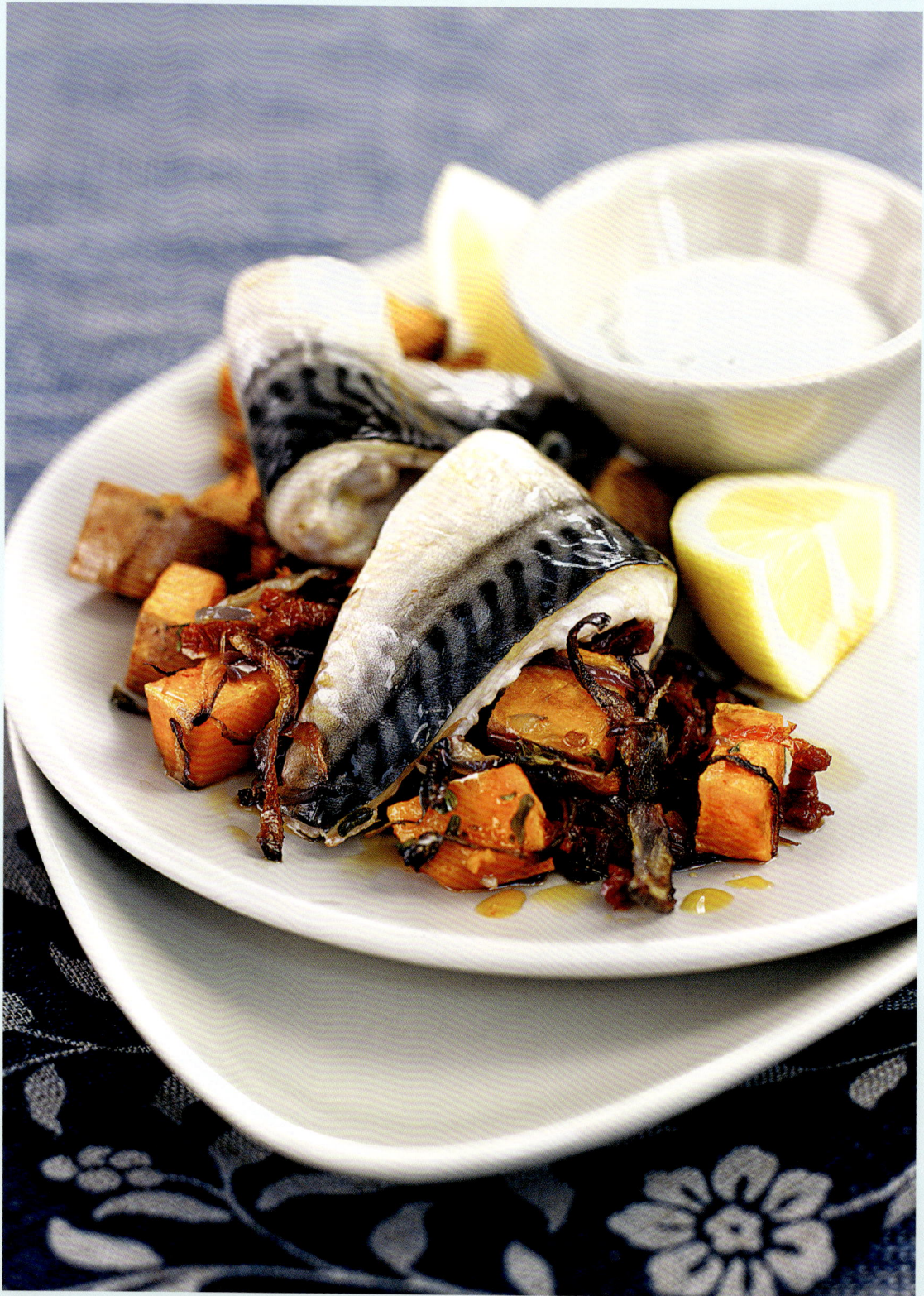

Mackerel
with Sweet Potatoes

Pair omega-3-rich mackerel with sweet potato, which contains the antioxidant beta-carotene and lots of fibre, to help keep blood sugar levels stable. Some find that due to the natural sweetness, sweet potato may even help to reduce any after-dinner sugar cravings.

SERVES **2**

375 g (12 oz) sweet potatoes, scrubbed and cut into 1.5-cm (¾-inch) chunks
1 red onion, thinly sliced
4 tablespoons chilli oil
several thyme sprigs
40 g (1½ oz) sun-dried tomatoes in oil, drained and thinly sliced
4 large mackerel fillets, pin-boned
100 ml (3½ fl oz) natural yogurt
1 tablespoon each chopped coriander and mint
salt and pepper
lemon wedges, to serve

1 Scatter the chunks of sweet potato in a shallow, ovenproof dish with the onion. Add the oil, thyme and a little salt and mix together.

2 Bake in a preheated oven, 200°C (400°F), Gas Mark 6, for 40–45 minutes, turning once or twice, until the potatoes are just tender and beginning to brown.

3 Stir in the tomatoes. Fold each mackerel fillet in half, skin-side out, and place on top of the potatoes. Return to the oven for a further 12–15 minutes, or until the fish is cooked through.

4 Meanwhile, mix together the yogurt, herbs and a little salt and pepper to make a raita. Transfer the fish and potatoes to warm plates, spoon over the raita and serve with lemon wedges.

Trout
with Pesto

If you're bored of salmon, try trout! It has a similar texture and is often more cost-effective. Pair with homemade pesto to elevate both the flavour and nutrition of the dish. Making pesto from scratch and storing it in the refrigerator is one of the easiest ways to liven up any dish in a matter of seconds. Plus, you've also added a serving of healthy fats.

SERVES **4**

4 tablespoons olive oil, plus extra
    for greasing
4 trout fillets, about 200 g (7 oz) each
large handful of basil, roughly chopped,
    plus extra to garnish
1 garlic clove, crushed
50 g (2 oz) Parmesan cheese,
    freshly grated
salt and pepper
salad, to serve

1   Brush a baking sheet lightly with oil and place under a preheated very hot grill to heat up.

2   Put the trout fillets on to the hot sheet, sprinkle with salt and pepper and place under the grill for 8–10 minutes until lightly browned and the fish flakes easily when pressed with a knife.

3   Meanwhile, put the basil and garlic into a bowl. Work in the oil using a hand-held blender. Stir in the Parmesan.

4   Remove the fish from the grill, transfer to serving plates, drizzle with the pesto, sprinkle with extra basil leaves to garnish and serve with salad.

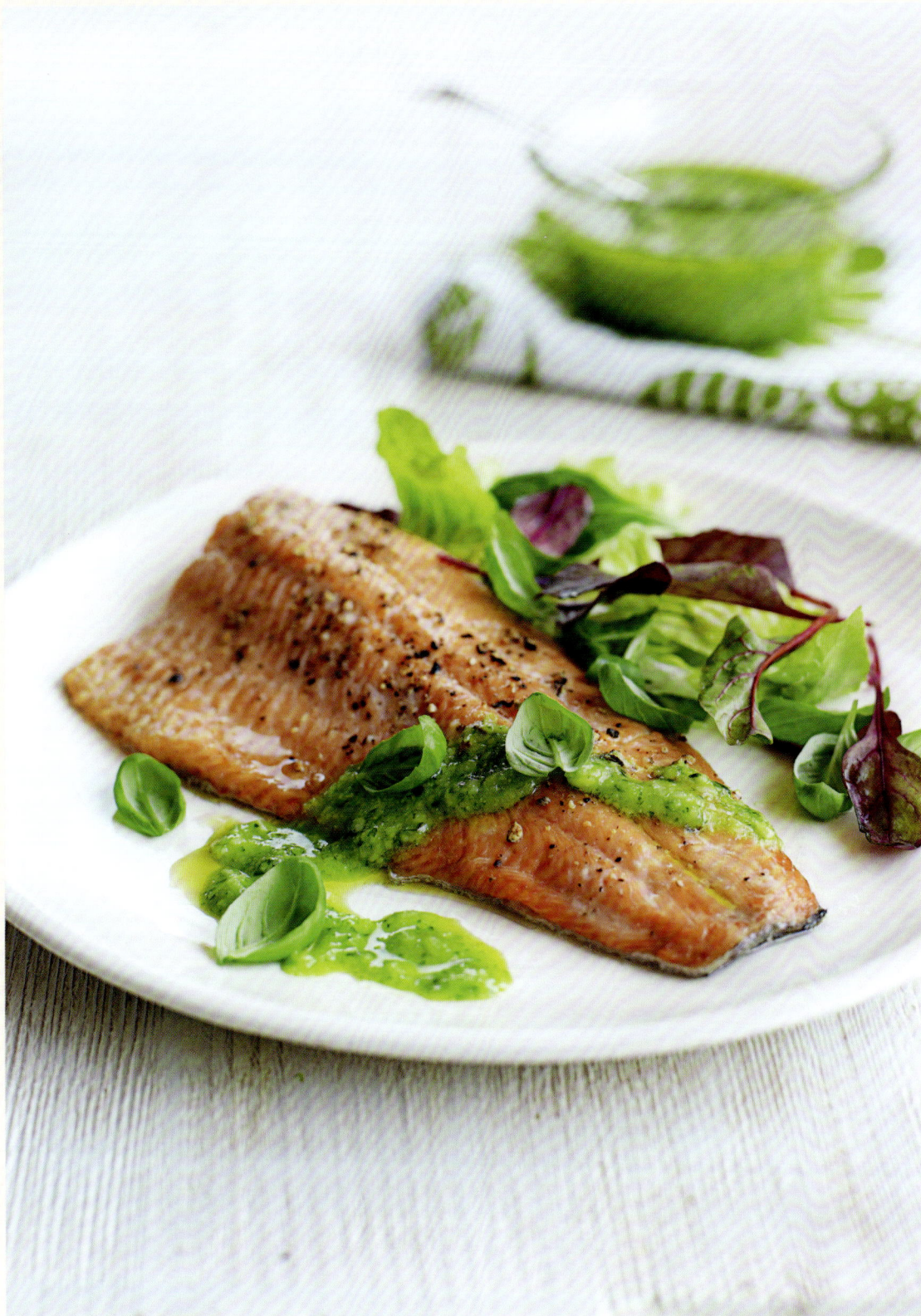

Salmon & Bulgur Wheat Pilaf

This is the type of recipe that shines when you're short on time midweek and need something quick, easy and nutritious for dinner. It is full of flavour from the fresh herbs and citrus, and contains all three macronutrients, meaning it'll keep blood sugar levels stable, helping you to manage PCOS symptoms.

SERVES 4

475 g (15 oz) boneless, skinless salmon
250 g (8 oz) bulgur wheat
75 g (3 oz) frozen peas
200 g (7 oz) runner beans, chopped
2 tablespoons chopped chives
2 tablespoons chopped flat leaf parsley
salt and pepper

TO SERVE

lemon wedges
natural yogurt

1 Cook the salmon in a steamer or microwave for about 10 minutes. Alternatively, wrap it in foil and cook in a preheated oven, 180°C (350°F), Gas Mark 4, for 15 minutes.

2 Meanwhile, cook the bulgur wheat according to the instructions on the packet and boil the peas and beans. Alternatively, cook the bulgur wheat, peas and beans in the steamer with the salmon.

3 Flake the salmon and mix it into the bulgur wheat with the peas and beans. Fold in the chives and parsley and season to taste. Serve immediately with lemon wedges and yogurt.

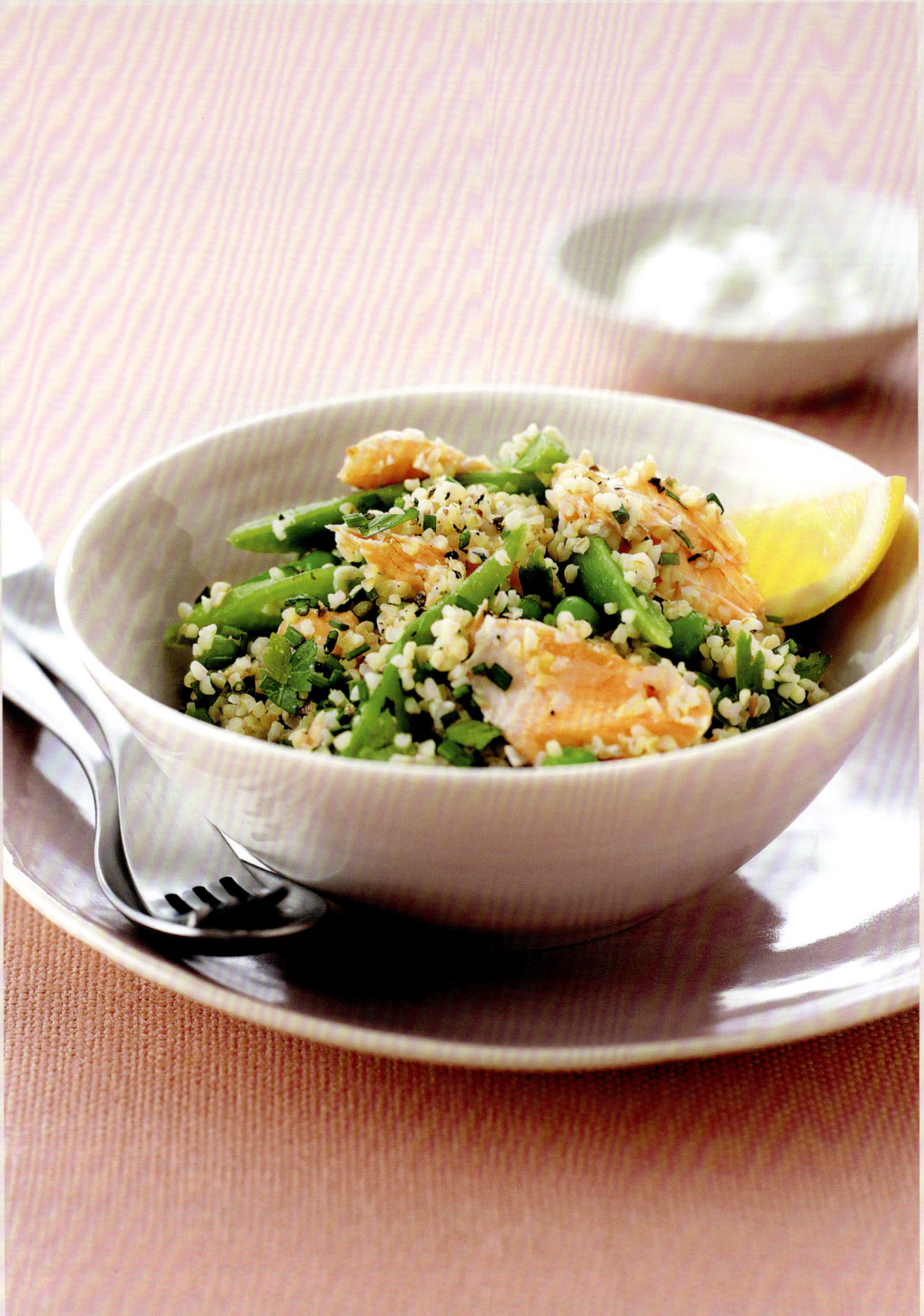

Chicken & Spinach Stew

Adding spinach or other dark leafy green vegetables is a great way to instantly boost the micronutrient profile of that meal and add extra fibre. Spinach contains magnesium, which contributes towards a healthy nervous system, as well as B vitamins, such as folate, which aids energy production.

SERVES **4**

625 g (1¼ lb) skinless, boneless chicken thighs, thinly sliced

2 teaspoons ground cumin

1 teaspoon ground ginger

2 tablespoons olive oil

1 tablespoon tomato purée

2 x 400 g (13 oz) cans cherry tomatoes

250 g (8 oz) cooked Puy lentils

1 teaspoon grated lemon zest

150 g (5 oz) baby spinach

salt and pepper

freshly chopped parsley, to garnish (optional)

steamed couscous or brown rice, to serve (optional)

1   Mix the chicken with the ground spices until well coated. Heat the olive oil in a large saucepan or flameproof casserole dish, then add the chicken and cook for 2–3 minutes, until lightly browned.

2   Stir in the tomato purée, tomatoes, lentils and lemon zest, season and simmer gently for about 12 minutes until thickened slightly and the chicken is cooked.

3   Add the spinach and stir until wilted.

4   Ladle the stew into bowls, then scatter with parsley and serve with steamed couscous or rice, if desired.

tip | Add a dollop of natural yogurt on top of this stew for a dose of probiotics, calcium and extra protein.

King Prawn & Sweet Potato Curry

Shellfish, including prawns, are a great source of zinc and selenium, two PCOS-healthy minerals. Zinc helps to regulate androgen levels and lowers insulin, while selenium has antioxidant properties that helps protects cells from damage.

SERVES 4

2 tablespoons olive oil

1 large onion, chopped

2 garlic cloves, sliced

1 tablespoon peeled and chopped fresh
　　root ginger

1 green chilli, thinly sliced

3 tablespoons mild curry paste

400 g (13 oz) sweet potato, diced

400 ml (14 fl oz) coconut milk

250 ml (8 fl oz) vegetable stock

small handful of curry leaves

400 g (13 oz) king prawns

100 g (3½ oz) frozen leaf spinach,
　　defrosted and drained

TO SERVE

brown rice

coriander leaves, freshly chopped

1　Heat the oil in a large, deep-sided frying pan or wok. Add the onion and cook over a medium-high heat for 3–4 minutes until beginning to colour. Add the garlic, ginger and chilli and stir-fry for a further 2 minutes. Reduce the heat slightly and add the curry paste, stirring for 1–2 minutes.

2　Add the sweet potato dice, tossing them to coat, then add the coconut milk, stock and curry leaves. Simmer gently for 12–15 minutes until the sweet potato is almost tender.

3　Add the prawns and spinach and stir over the heat for 2–3 minutes until the prawns are just cooked through.

4　Spoon the curry into dishes and serve immediately with brown rice and chopped coriander.

tip | No prawns on hand? Salmon is a great substitute in this recipe.

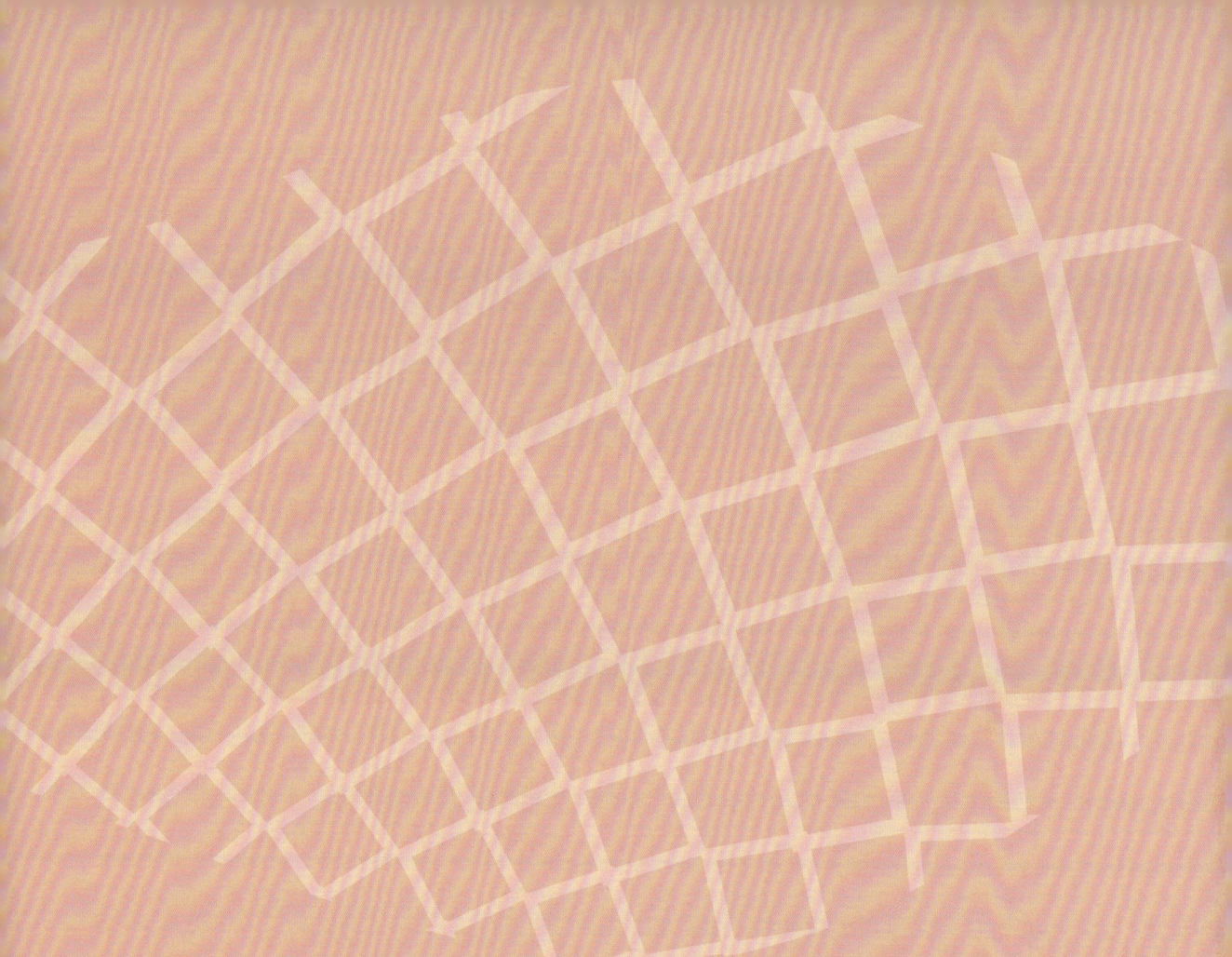

Sweet Treats
& Desserts

Oaty Raspberry Dessert

Who says oats should be reserved for breakfast? When creating delicious desserts to help manage PCOS symptoms, boosting the fibre content and opting for low-sugar fruits is a great way to prevent blood sugar spikes that often follow high-sugar dishes. The oats and berries in this dessert do just that, providing natural sweetness while helping you feel your best.

SERVES 4

100 g (3½ oz) rolled oats

50 g (2 oz) heather honey, plus extra
    to serve

300 ml (½ pint) Greek yogurt

225 g (7½ oz) raspberries

1   Place the oats on a baking sheet, drizzle with the honey and stir around a little. Toast under a preheated medium grill for about 6–8 minutes, turning occasionally, until golden, watching carefully to ensure they do not burn. Transfer to a plate to cool slightly.

2   Gently mix together the toasted oats, yogurt and raspberries in a bowl until just combined – do not over-mix.

3   Divide between 4 small bowls or glasses and serve drizzled with extra honey.

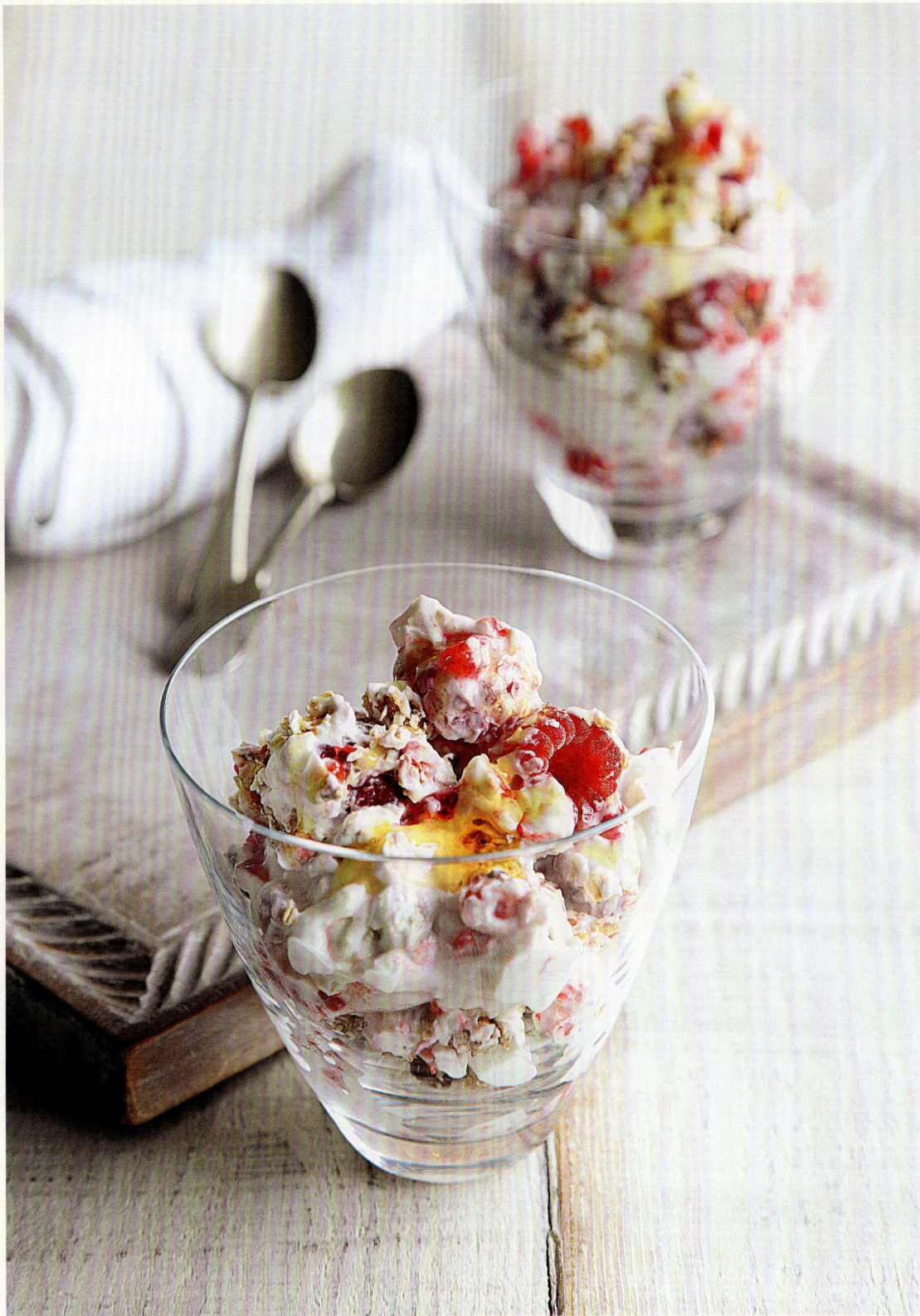

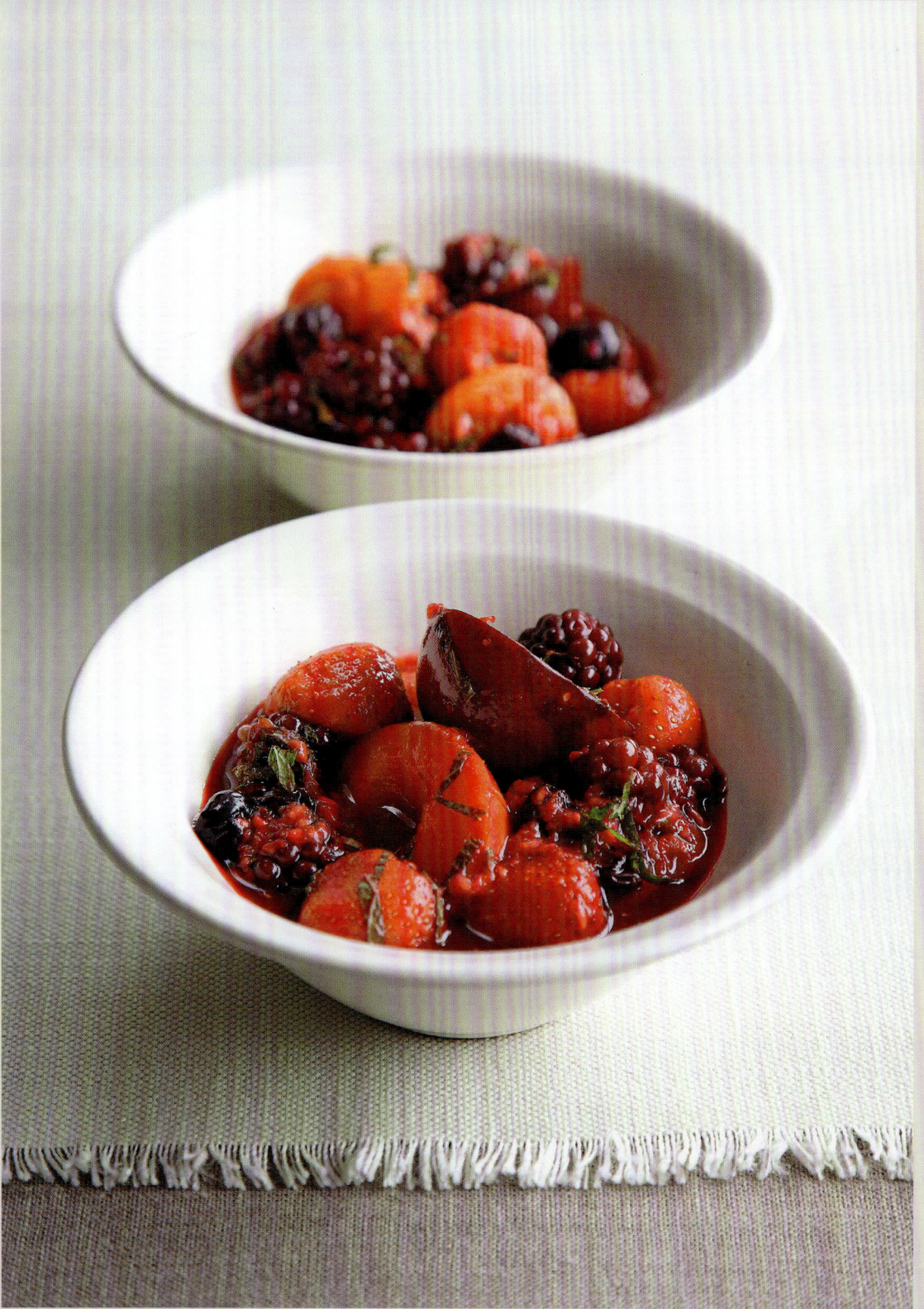

Berry & Mint Compôte

This vibrant berry compôte is rich in polyphenols, antioxidants that are great for your skin and contribute to a healthy gut microbiome. Polyphenols also help to reduce systemic inflammation, which can drive a number of PCOS symptoms. It is a great way to liven up your yogurt!

SERVES 4

450 g (14½ oz) mixed fruit, such
    as strawberries, blackberries,
    raspberries, and halved and
    stoned plums
1 cinnamon stick
grated zest and juice of 1 orange
8 mint leaves, shredded
natural yogurt, to serve (optional)

1   Place the fruit, cinnamon stick and orange zest and juice in a small saucepan and simmer gently for 12–15 minutes.

2   Remove the cinnamon stick, leave the compôte to cool for 3–4 minutes, then stir in the mint.

3   Serve with dollops of natural yogurt, if liked.

Baked Spiced Bananas

In need of something sweet but speedy after your meal? These baked bananas might just be your new go-to! Bananas contain tryptophan, an amino acid that your body converts into serotonin and melatonin, and vitamin B6 which facilitates this conversion. A dollop of yogurt provides both protein and probiotics, supporting blood sugar levels and your gut microbiome.

SERVES **4**

4 ripe bananas, sliced lengthways
butter, for greasing
1 teaspoon ground allspice
½ teaspoon ground nutmeg
juice of 1 lemon
50 g (2 oz) flaked almonds
3 knobs of stem ginger, diced
200 g (7 oz) natural yogurt

1   Place the bananas in a lightly greased ovenproof dish. Sprinkle over the spices, lemon juice and almonds.

2   Bake in a preheated oven, 180°C (350°F), Gas Mark 4, for 12–15 minutes.

3   Meanwhile, mix together the stem ginger and yogurt in a bowl.

4   Serve the bananas with dollops of the yogurt on top.

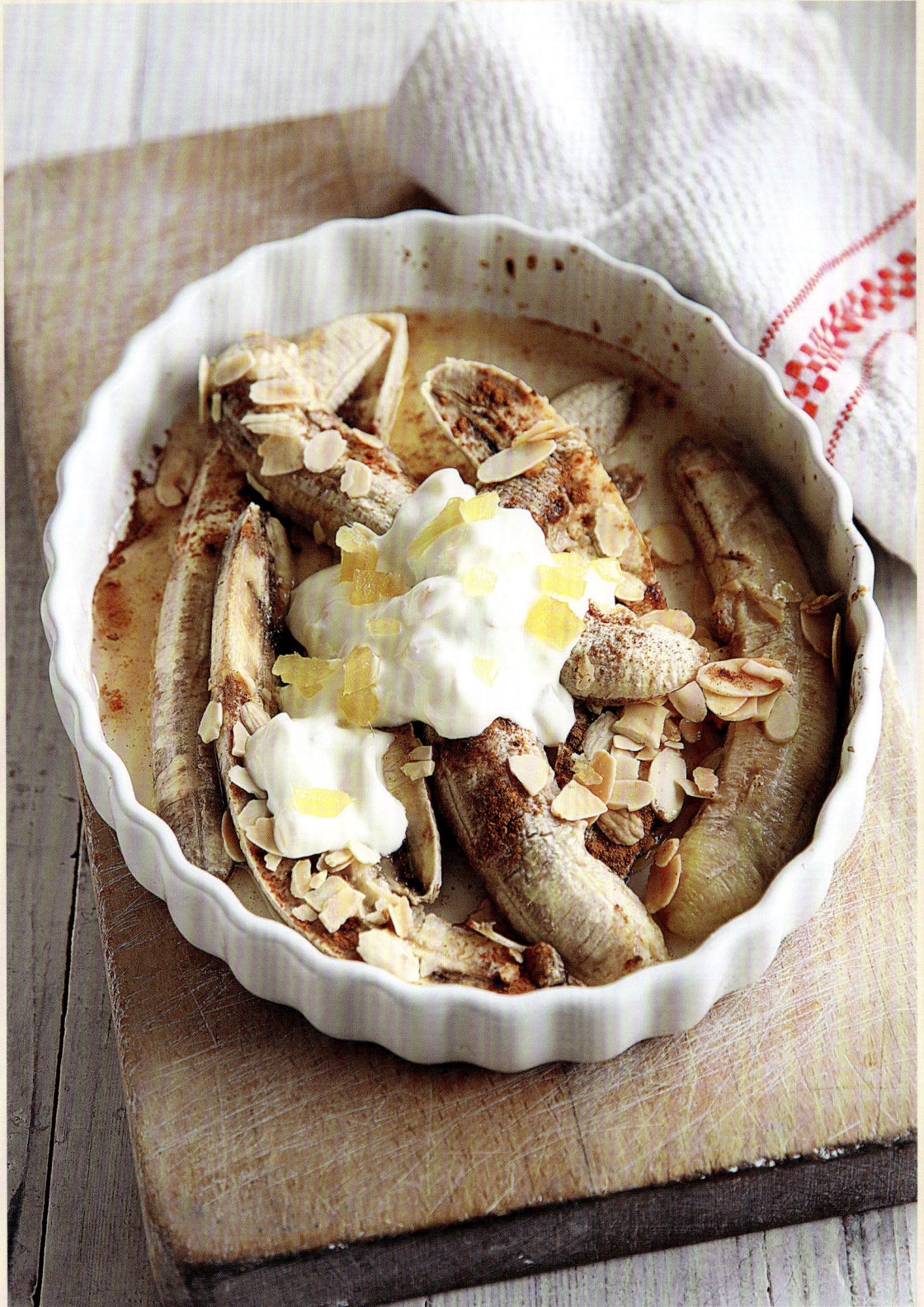

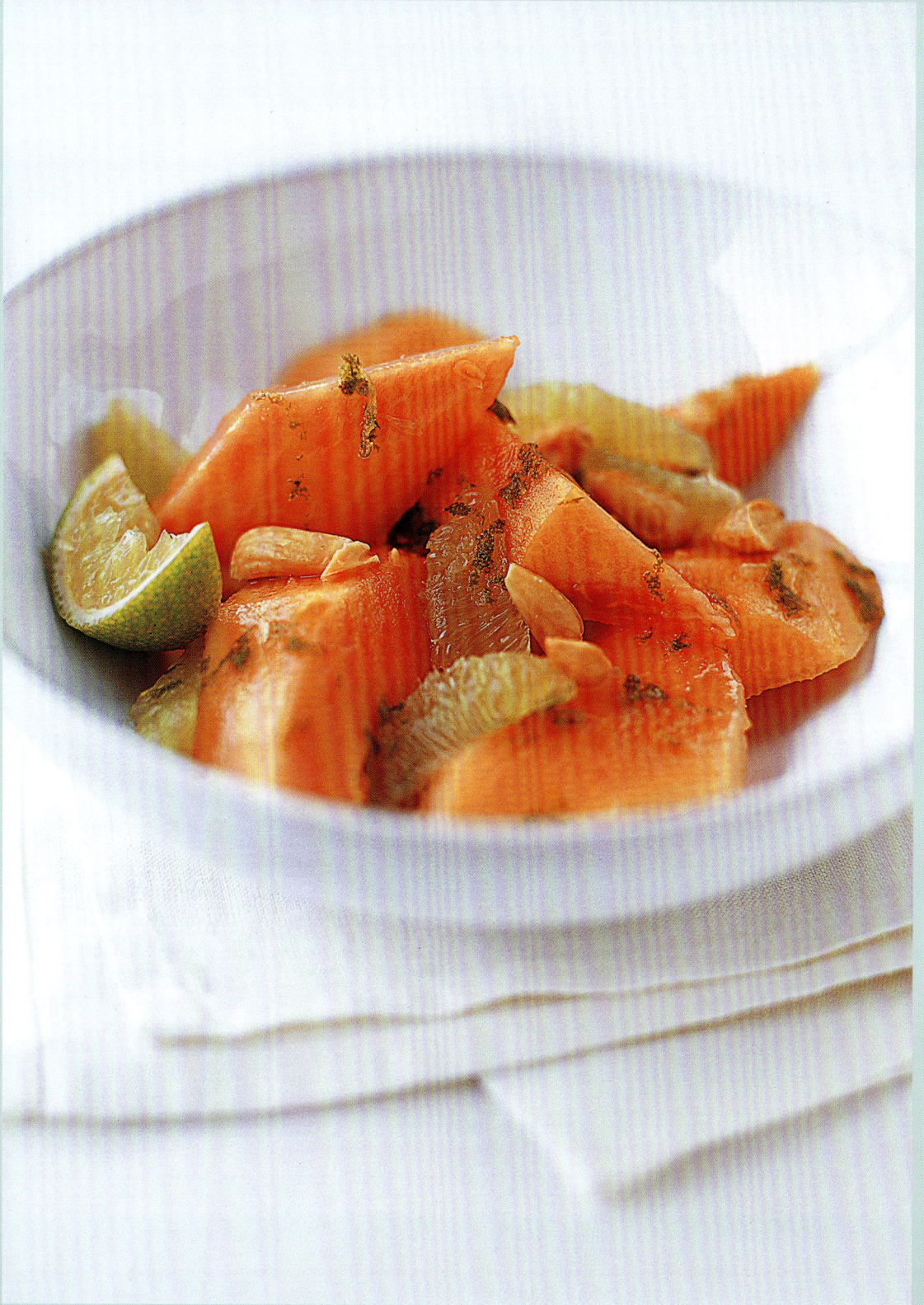

Papaya, Lime & Almond Salad

Papaya contains a digestive enzyme called papain, which helps with the digestion of protein. Including papaya in a dessert such as this, where it is muddled with lime and almonds, is a great way to support your digestion. Both papaya and lime are rich in vitamin C, which has antioxidant properties, reducing oxidative stress.

SERVES 4

3 firm, ripe papayas, peeled and deseeded
2 limes
50 g (2 oz) toasted blanched almonds
lime wedges, to decorate

1   Cut the papayas into large dice.

2   Finely grate the zest of both limes, then squeeze 1 of the limes and reserve the juice. Cut the pith off the second lime and segment the flesh over the bowl of papaya to catch the juice. Add the lime segments and grated zest to the bowl.

3   Pour the reserved lime juice over the fruit and toss thoroughly. Add the toasted almonds and serve with lime wedges.

tip | A dollop of natural or Greek yogurt makes a great accompaniment to this recipe!

Baked Figs
with Yogurt

We often think of berries as being loaded with antioxidants, but did you know figs are another great source? They contain polyphenols, plant compounds with antioxidant properties, making them great for cardiovascular and metabolic health. Figs are packed full of fibre too, and eaten alongside high-protein Greek yogurt helps to stabilize their natural sugars.

SERVES 4

8 fresh figs, rinsed in cold water

about 3 teaspoons rosewater

2 tablespoons runny honey

50 g (2 oz) unsalted butter

250 g (8 oz) Greek yogurt

small handful of walnuts,
    roughly chopped

1   Cut a cross in the top of each fig and open out the cut to halfway through the fruit. Arrange the figs in a small roasting tin or shallow ovenproof dish. Add a few drops of rosewater to each fig, then drizzle with 1½ tablespoons of the honey and dot with the butter. Bake in a preheated oven, 190°C (375°F), Gas Mark 5, for 8–10 minutes until the figs are hot but still firm.

2   Meanwhile, mix the yogurt with the remaining honey and gradually mix in a little of the remaining rosewater to taste.

3   Transfer the figs to shallow serving dishes and serve with spoonfuls of yogurt, sprinkled with chopped walnuts.

Honey-roasted Peaches

Keeping refined sugars on the lower end can be tough at times, especially when many desserts are designed to be highly palatable. Having a number of nutritious and well-balanced sweet alternatives up your sleeve is a great way to satisfy your sweet tooth without jumping on the blood sugar rollercoaster. Peaches are packed full of polyphenols, carotenoids and vitamin C, all helping to reduce oxidative stress and support metabolic health.

SERVES 4

2 tablespoons orange blossom honey
1 vanilla pod, split lengthways
2–3 teaspoons sesame seeds
4 peaches, halved and stoned
Greek yogurt, to serve

1 Pour the honey into a small saucepan. Scrape the seeds from the vanilla pod and add the seeds and pod to the pan. Heat gently, stirring occasionally. Stir in the sesame seeds.

2 Place the peaches in a roasting tin and pour over the honey mixture. Bake in a preheated oven, 180°C (350°F), Gas Mark 4, for 20–25 minutes until the peaches are soft. Baste a couple of times with the juices.

3 Serve warm with Greek yogurt.

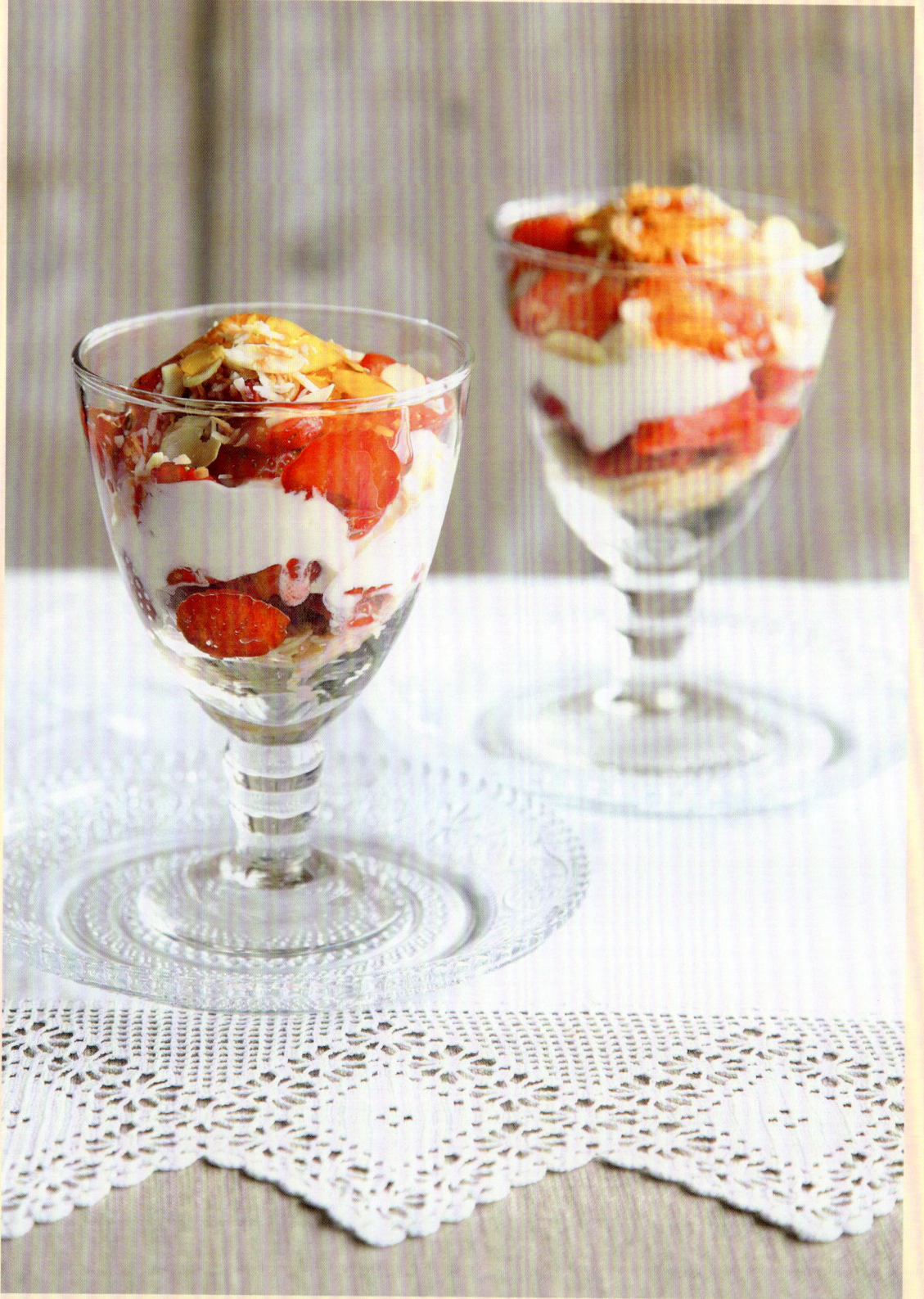

Strawberry & Almond Desserts

If you love the flavour of strawberries and cream, this is the recipe for you! Strawberries are a great PCOS-friendly fruit due to their high fibre and low sugar content, as well as being rich in vitamin C.

SERVES **4**

4 tablespoons flaked almonds
4 tablespoons desiccated coconut
300 g (10 oz) strawberries, hulled and sliced
250 g (8 oz) natural yogurt
2 teaspoons clear honey

1   Place the flaked almonds and coconut on a baking sheet and cook under a preheated medium-hot grill for 3–4 minutes until golden, turning at least once. Leave to cool.

2   Spoon half of the almond and coconut mixture into 4 glasses. Layer with half of the sliced strawberries, then the yogurt.

3   Top with the remaining strawberries, almonds and coconut. Spoon over the honey and serve.

tip | No strawberries on hand? Any other berry will work great here too.

Honeyed Ricotta
with Summer Fruits

Because cheese contains a good amount of protein and fat, it makes for a PCOS-friendly dessert option. Whether you have it as a savoury dish, or sweetened with berries and honey as demonstrated in this recipe, your glucose levels will feel stable, which is key in managing your symptoms.

SERVES **4**

125 g (4 oz) fresh raspberries

2 teaspoons rosewater

250 g (8 oz) ricotta cheese

250 g (8 oz) fresh mixed summer
    berries

2 tablespoons clear honey with
    honeycomb

2 tablespoons pumpkin seeds, toasted

pinch of ground cinnamon

1   Rub the raspberries through a fine nylon sieve to purée and remove the pips, then mix with the rosewater. Alternatively, put the raspberries and rosewater in a food processor or blender and process to a purée, then sieve to remove the pips.

2   Slice the ricotta into wedges and arrange on serving plates with the berries. Drizzle over the honey and the raspberry purée, adding a little honeycomb, and serve sprinkled with the pumpkin seeds and cinnamon.

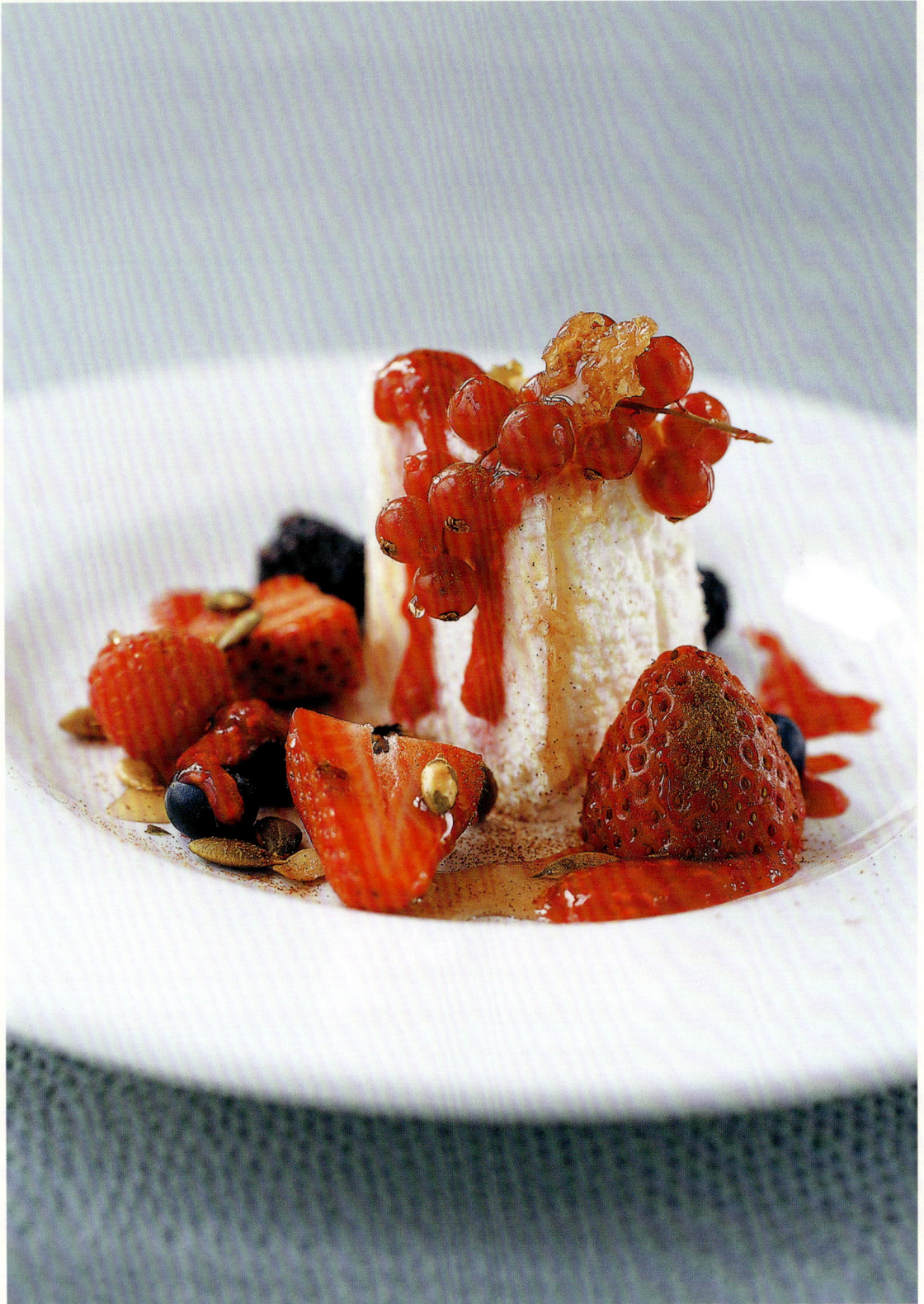

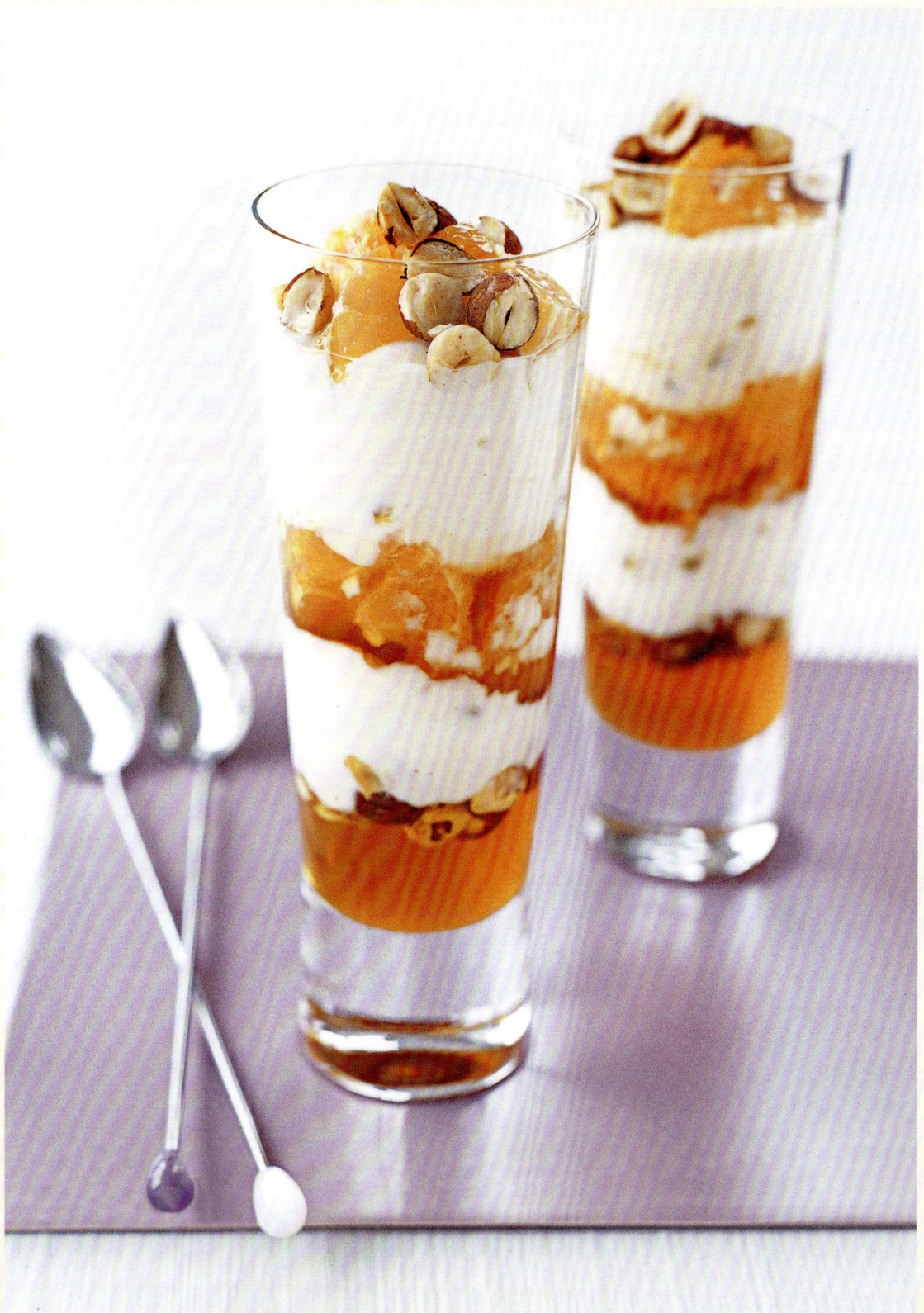

Nutty Passion Fruit Yogurts

If you're looking for a way to liven up plain yogurt, passion fruit is a great way to do just that. It takes seconds to scoop out of its thick skin, and adds tang, texture and juice. Yogurt contains a vast amount of probiotic strains to help maintain the healthy bacteria in your gut, contributing to a balanced mood and immune system.

SERVES **2**

2 passion fruit

250 ml (8 fl oz) natural yogurt

2 tablespoons clear honey

50 g (2 oz) hazelnuts, toasted and
 roughly chopped

4 clementines, peeled and chopped
 into small pieces

1   Halve the passion fruit and scoop the pulp into a large bowl. Add the yogurt and mix them together gently.

2   Divide 1 tablespoon of the honey between the bases of two narrow glasses and scatter with half of the hazelnuts. Spoon half of the yogurt mixture over the nuts and arrange half of the clementine pieces on top of the yogurt.

3   Repeat the layering, reserving a few of the nuts for decoration. Scatter the nuts over the top and chill the yogurts until you are ready to serve them.

Chocolate Pots

Craving something sweet and chocolatey after your meal? These individual chocolate pots are a great choice. By having something sweet as a dessert rather than on its own, you reduce the intensity of the blood sugar spike. What's more, cacao is a great source of antioxidants and provides an instant mood boost.

SERVES **4**

50 g (2 oz) melted butter, plus extra
    for greasing
75 g (3 oz) plain flour
1 teaspoon baking powder
1 tablespoon cacao powder
25 g (1 oz) ground almonds
50 g (2 oz) coconut sugar
1 egg, lightly beaten
50 ml (2 fl oz) semi-skimmed milk
125 g (4 oz) raspberries, to serve

1   Preheat the oven to 180°C (350°F), Gas Mark 4. Lightly grease 4 mini pudding basins, 175 ml (6 fl oz) each. Sift together the flour, baking powder and cacao powder into a bowl. Stir in the ground almonds and coconut sugar.

2   Beat the egg with the milk and melted butter in a small bowl, then pour into the dry ingredients and stir until combined.

3   Spoon the mixture into the prepared pudding basins and bake in the oven for 15 minutes, or until risen and firm to the touch.

4   Serve the chocolate pots warm with fresh raspberries.

tip | Add a dollop of yogurt on top for a helping of healthy fats and extra protein!

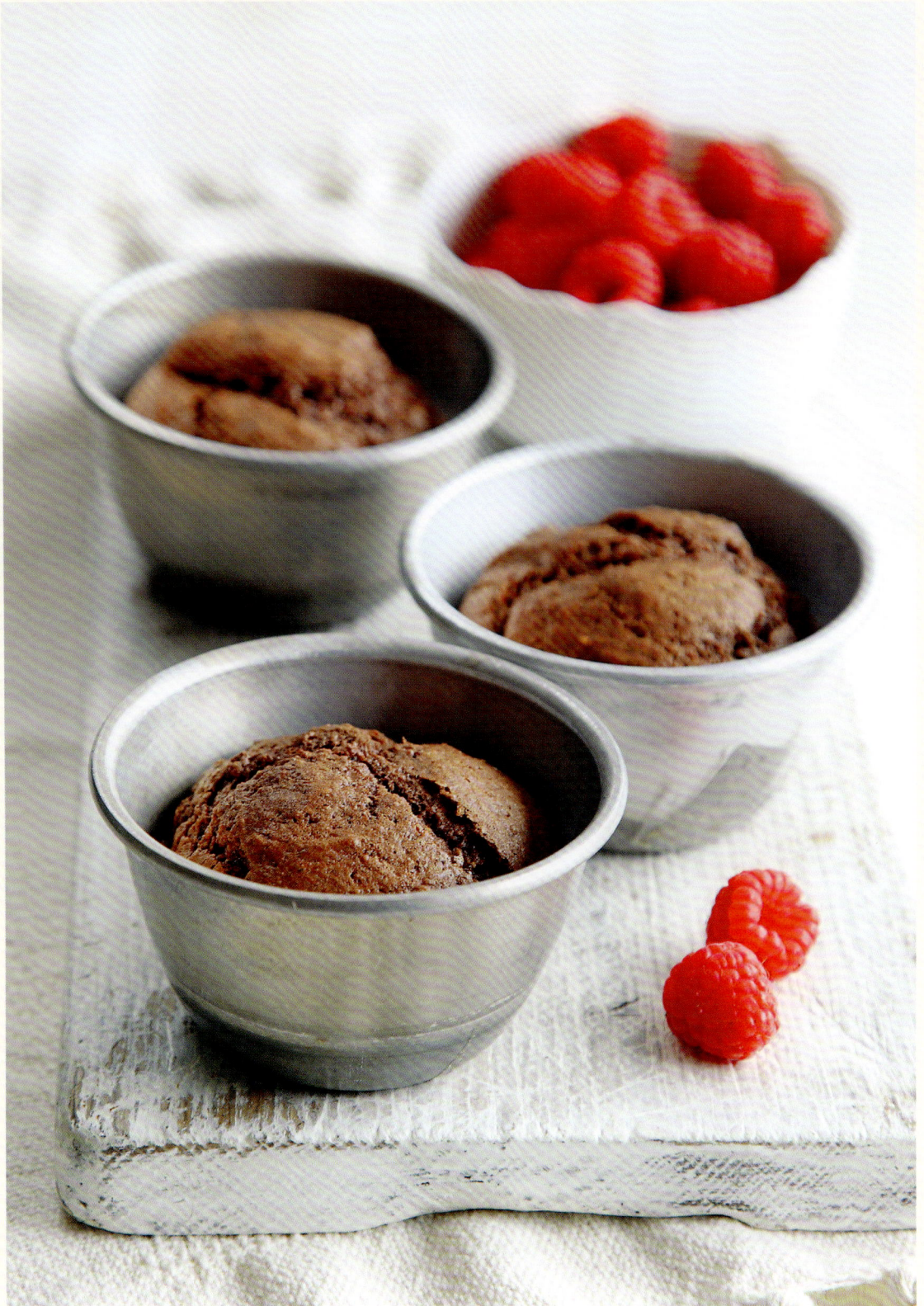

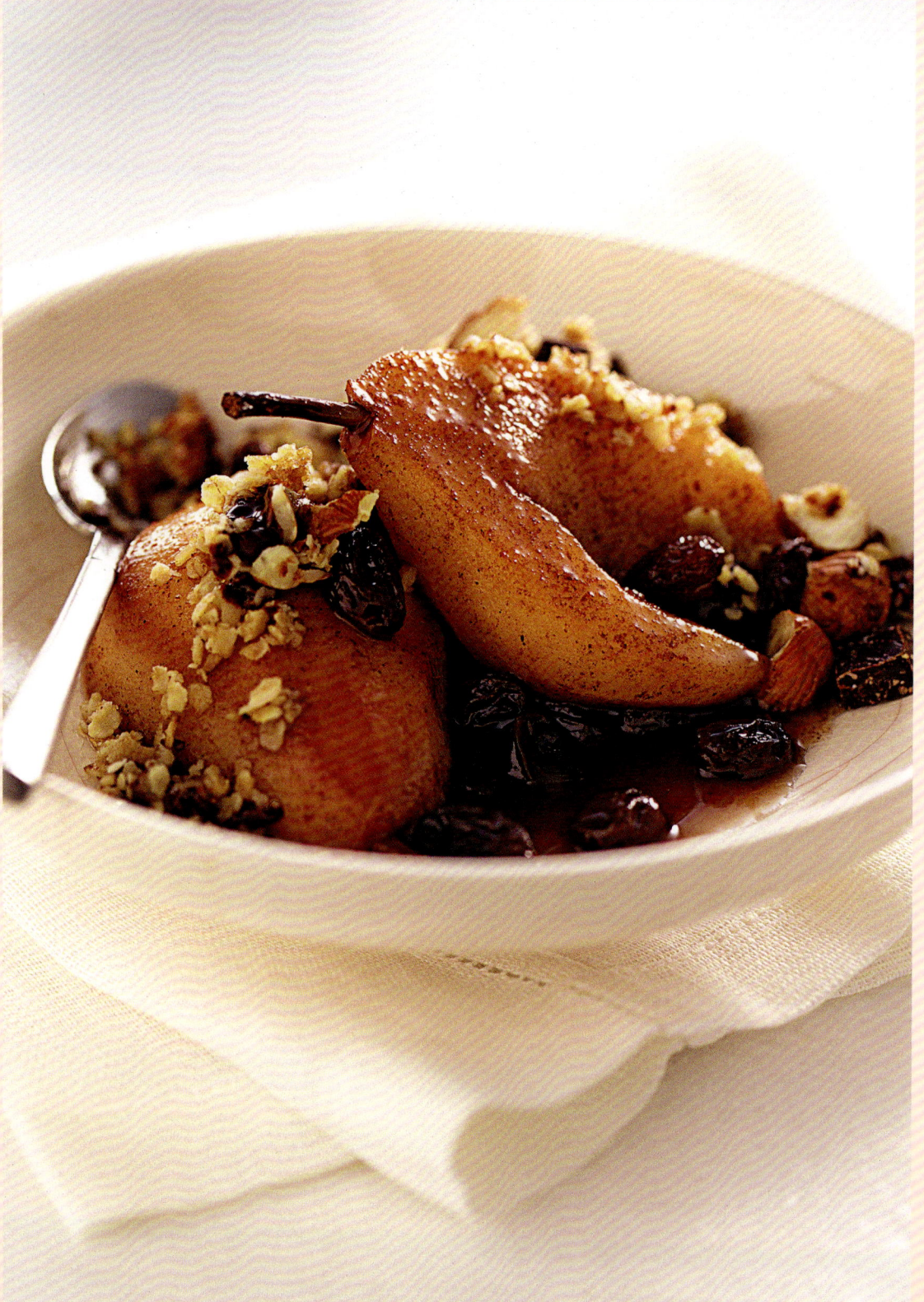

Pears
with Chocolate Crumble

Pears are rich in insoluble fibre, specifically pectin, which is highly beneficial for the gut microbiome. The chocolate crumble sprinkled over the top adds a lovely additional layer of texture and flavour against the pears, while providing an extra hit of polyphenols.

SERVES 4

25 g (1 oz) coconut sugar

150 ml (¼ pint) water

25 g (1 oz) raisins

½ teaspoon ground cinnamon

4 ripe dessert pears, peeled, halved
    and cored

40 g (1½ oz) unsalted butter

50 g (2 oz) porridge oats

25 g (1 oz) hazelnuts, roughly chopped

50 g (2 oz) plain chocolate or milk
    chocolate, chopped

lightly whipped cream or Greek yogurt,
    to serve (optional)

1   Place half of the sugar in a frying pan or wide sauté pan with the measured water and the raisins and cinnamon. Bring just to the boil, then add the pears and simmer gently, uncovered, for about 5 minutes until the pears are slightly softened.

2   Melt the butter in a separate frying pan or saucepan. Add the porridge oats and fry gently for 2 minutes. Stir in the remaining sugar and cook over a gentle heat until golden.

3   Spoon the pears on to serving plates. Stir the hazelnuts and chocolate into the oat mixture. Once the chocolate starts to melt, spoon over the pears. Serve topped with whipped cream or Greek yogurt, if liked.

tip | This recipe would also work with apples and is a great way to use up the fruit you have left over in your fruit bowl.

Fruit Granola Bars

Using high-fibre staples, such as fresh fruit and dates, is a great way to sweeten your desserts and keep blood glucose levels stable. Flaxseed and oats provide two extra prebiotic fibre sources to keep the good bugs in your gut, while peanut butter gives these bars a lovely nutty flavour and healthy fats at the same time.

MAKES **9**

225 g (7½ oz) peeled, cored and
    roughly chopped dessert apple
1 tablespoon lemon juice
1 tablespoon maple syrup
½ teaspoon ground cinnamon
olive oil, for oiling

GRANOLA

125 g (4 oz) rolled oats
125 g (4 oz) ready-to-eat dried apricots
125 g (4 oz) fresh Medjool dates,
    stoned and roughly chopped
2 tablespoons ground flaxseed (linseed)
2 tablespoons smooth peanut butter
55 ml (2 fl oz) agave syrup

1   Line a baking sheet with baking parchment. Toss the apple with the lemon juice, maple syrup and cinnamon in a bowl, then spread out on the lined baking sheet and roast in a preheated oven, 160°C (325°F), Gas Mark 3, for 20 minutes. Remove from the oven and leave to cool.

2   Increase the oven temperature to 180°C (350°F), Gas Mark 4. Pulse all the ingredients for the granola together in a food processor a few times until mixed and mashed. Fold in the cooled roasted apple, then spoon into a lightly oiled 20 cm (8 inch) square shallow cake tin and level with the back of a spoon. Bake in the oven for 20 minutes.

3   Leave to cool for 15 minutes before cutting into 9 squares to serve.

tip | Not a fan of peanut butter? Swap it for almond butter or tahini.

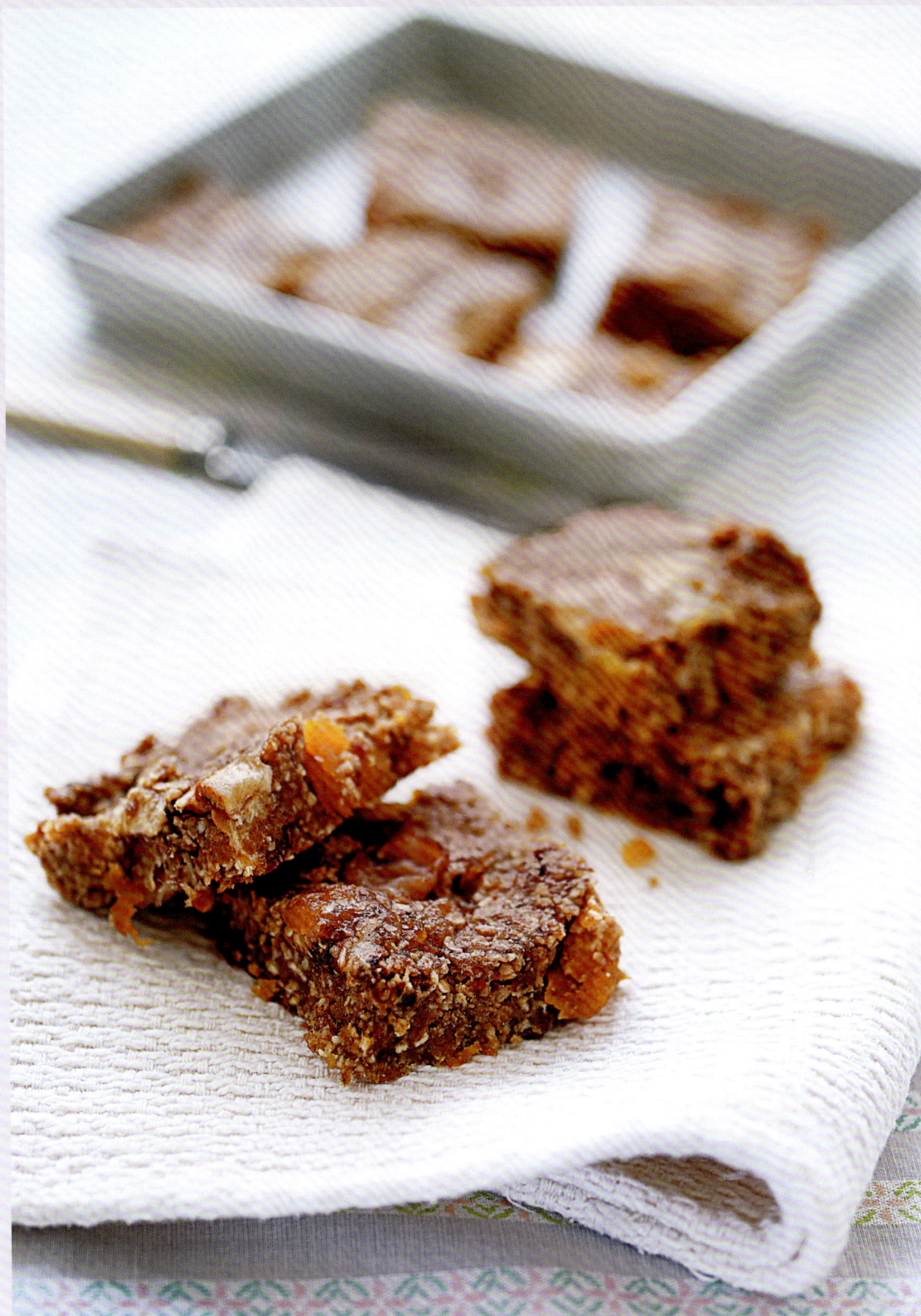

References

INTRODUCTION

4 'environmental toxins': Christ, J. P., & Cedars, M. I. (2023). Current Guidelines for Diagnosing PCOS. *Diagnostics* (Basel, Switzerland), 13(6), 1113. https://doi.org/10.3390/diagnostics13061113

4 'exposure to androgens in the womb': Filippou, P., & Homburg, R. (2017). Is foetal hyperexposure to androgens a cause of PCOS?. *Human Reproduction Update*, 23(4), 421–432. https://doi.org/10.1093/humupd/dmx013

4 'Eating a healthy, well-balanced diet has been shown to improve some symptoms': https://www.nhs.uk/conditions/polycystic-ovary-syndrome-pcos/

5 'this is behind many of the symptoms we now associate with PCOS': Singh, S., Pal, N., Shubham, S., Sarma, D. K., Verma, V., Marotta, F., & Kumar, M. (2023). Polycystic Ovary Syndrome: Etiology, Current Management, and Future Therapeutics. *Journal of Clinical Medicine*, 12(4), 1454. https://doi.org/10.3390/jcm12041454

5 'raised insulin drives excess androgens': Ding, H., Zhang, J., Zhang, F., Zhang, S., Chen, X., Liang, W., & Xie, Q. (2021). Resistance to the Insulin and Elevated Level of Androgen: A Major Cause of Polycystic Ovary Syndrome. *Frontiers in Endocrinology*, 12, 741764. https://doi.org/10.3389/fendo.2021.741764

5 'our cells are unable to take in as much glucose': Singh, S. et al. (2023). Polycystic Ovary Syndrome.

5 'Insulin increases androgens': Ibid.

5 'The less SHBG, the more free testosterone roaming around the body': Xing, C., Zhang, J., Zhao, H., & He, B. (2022). Effect of Sex Hormone-Binding Globulin on Polycystic Ovary Syndrome: Mechanisms, Manifestations, Genetics, and Treatment. *International Journal of Women's Health*, 14, 91–105. https://doi.org/10.2147/IJWH.S344542

6 'high testosterone also increases insulin resistance': Singh, S. et al. (2023). Polycystic Ovary Syndrome.

6 'Androgen Excess Society (AES) argued that hyperandrogenism should be essential in diagnosing PCOS': Azziz, R., Carmina, E., Dewailly, D., Diamanti-Kandarakis, E., Escobar-Morreale, H. F., Futterweit, W., Janssen, O. E., Legro, R. S., Norman, R. J., Taylor, A. E., Witchel, S. F., & Task Force on the Phenotype of the Polycystic Ovary Syndrome of The Androgen Excess and PCOS Society (2009). The Androgen Excess and PCOS Society criteria for the polycystic ovary syndrome: the complete task force report. *Fertility and Sterility*, 91(2), 456–488. https://doi.org/10.1016/j.fertnstert.2008.06.035

7 'those with PCOS may present with higher levels of AMH': Butt, M. S., Saleem, J., Aiman, S., Zakar, R., Sadique, I., & Fischer, F. (2022). Serum anti-Müllerian hormone as a predictor of polycystic ovarian syndrome among women of reproductive age. *BMC Women's Health*, 22(1), 199. https://doi.org/10.1186/s12905-022-01782-2

8 'may increase complications during pregnancy': Yu, H. F., Chen, H. S., Rao, D. P., & Gong, J. (2016). Association between polycystic ovary syndrome and the risk of pregnancy complications: A PRISMA-compliant systematic review and meta-analysis. *Medicine*, 95(51), e4863. https://doi.org/10.1097/MD.0000000000004863

8 'increased risk of endometrial cancer': Johnson, J. E., Daley, D., Tarta, C., & Stanciu, P. I. (2023). Risk of endometrial cancer in patients with polycystic ovarian syndrome: A meta-analysis. *Oncology Letters*, 25(4), 168. https://doi.org/10.3892/ol.2023.13754

8 'more likely to experience mental health issues, such as eating disorders, depression': Himelein, M. J., & Thatcher, S. S. (2006). Depression and body image among women with polycystic ovary syndrome. *Journal of Health Psychology*, 11(4), 613–625. https://doi.org/10.1177/1359105306065021

8 'more likely to experience mental health issues, such as [...] depression and anxiety': Dokras A. (2012). Mood and anxiety disorders in women with PCOS. *Steroids*, 77(4), 338–341. https://doi.org/10.1016/j.steroids.2011.12.008

8 'helping to regulate insulin production and blood glucose levels': Shang, Y., Zhou, H., Hu, M., & Feng, H. (2020). Effect of Diet on Insulin Resistance in Polycystic Ovary Syndrome. *The Journal of clinical endocrinology and metabolism*, 105(10), dgaa425. https://doi.org/10.1210/clinem/dgaa425

9 'it can help to keep carbohydrate consumption low': Zhang, X., Zheng, Y., Guo, Y., & Lai, Z. (2019). The Effect of Low Carbohydrate Diet on Polycystic Ovary Syndrome: A Meta-Analysis of Randomized Controlled Trials. *International Journal of Endocrinology*, 2019, 4386401. https://doi.org/10.1155/2019/4386401

9 'promising results with the keto diet': Khalid, K., Apparow, S., Mushaddik, I. L., Anuar, A., Rizvi, S. A. A., & Habib, A. (2023). Effects of Ketogenic Diet on Reproductive Hormones in Women With Polycystic Ovary Syndrome. *Journal of the Endocrine Society*, 7(10), bvad112. https://doi.org/10.1210/jendso/bvad112

9 'excess intake of simple carbohydrates and refined sugars worsens insulin resistance': Barrea, L., Marzullo, P., Muscogiuri, G., Di Somma, C., Scacchi, M., Orio, F., Aimaretti, G., Colao, A., & Savastano, S. (2018). Source and amount of carbohydrate in the diet and inflammation in women with polycystic ovary syndrome. *Nutrition Research Reviews*, 31(2), 291–301. https://doi.org/10.1017/S0954422418000136

9 'You can have insulin resistance and not experience weight gain or difficulty maintaining a healthy weight': Toosy, S., Sodi, R., & Pappachan, J. M. (2018). Lean polycystic ovary syndrome (PCOS): an evidence-based practical approach. *Journal of Diabetes and Metabolic Disorders*, 17(2), 277–285. https://doi.org/10.1007/s40200-018-0371-5

9 'do show an improvement in symptoms': Khalid, K., Apparow, S., Mushaddik, I. L., Anuar, A., Rizvi, S. A. A., & Habib, A. (2023). Effects of Ketogenic Diet on Reproductive Hormones in Women With Polycystic Ovary Syndrome. *Journal of the Endocrine Society*,

7(10), bvad112. https://doi.org/10.1210/jendso/bvad112

9 'do show an improvement in symptoms': Velissariou, M., Athanasiadou, C. R., Diamanti, A., Lykeridou, A., & Sarantaki, A. (2025). The impact of intermittent fasting on fertility: A focus on polycystic ovary syndrome and reproductive outcomes in Women-A systematic review. *Metabolism Open*, 25, 100341. https://doi.org/10.1016/j.metop.2024.100341

9 'shown to benefit weight loss': Cunha, N. B. D., Ribeiro, C. T., Silva, C. M., Rosa-E-Silva, A. C. J. S., & De-Souza, D. A. (2019). Dietary intake, body composition and metabolic parameters in women with polycystic ovary syndrome. *Clinical Nutrition* (Edinburgh, Scotland), 38(5), 2342–2348. https://doi.org/10.1016/j.clnu.2018.10.012

10 'muscle mass increases insulin sensitivity': Haines, M. S., Dichtel, L. E., Santoso, K., Torriani, M., Miller, K. K., & Bredella, M. A. (2020). Association between muscle mass and insulin sensitivity independent of detrimental adipose depots in young adults with overweight/obesity. *International Journal of Obesity* (2005), 44(9), 1851–1858. https://doi.org/10.1038/s41366-020-0590-y

11 'molecules in the oils can become unstable and problematic in the body': Ambreen, G., Siddiq, A., & Hussain, K. (2020). Association of long-term consumption of repeatedly heated mix vegetable oils in different doses and hepatic toxicity through fat accumulation. *Lipids in Health and Disease*, 19(1), 69. https://doi.org/10.1186/s12944-020-01256-0

11 'it may lower androgens and insulin levels': Melo, V., Silva, T., Silva, T., Freitas, J., Sacramento, J., Vazquez, M., & Araujo, E. (2022). Omega-3 supplementation in the treatment of polycystic ovary syndrome (PCOS) – a review of clinical trials and cohort. *Endocrine Regulations*, 56(1), 66–79. https://doi.org/10.2478/enr-2022-0008

11 'it may lower androgens and insulin levels': Albardan, L., Platat, C., & Kalupahana, N. S. (2024). Role of Omega-3 Fatty Acids in Improving Metabolic Dysfunctions in Polycystic Ovary Syndrome. *Nutrients*, 16(17), 2961. https://doi.org/10.3390/nu16172961

11 'Zinc […] supports the immune system, and can help to regulate androgens': Abedini, M., Ghaedi, E., Hadi, A., Mohammadi, H., & Amani, R. (2019). Zinc status and polycystic ovarian syndrome: A systematic review and meta-analysis. *Journal of Trace Elements in Medicine and Biology: organ of the Society for Minerals and Trace Elements* (GMS), 52, 216–221. https://doi.org/10.1016/j.jtemb.2019.01.002

12 'which is known to increase inflammation and complications related to PCOS': Li, W., Liu, C., Yang, Q., Zhou, Y., Liu, M., & Shan, H. (2022). Oxidative stress and antioxidant imbalance in ovulation disorder in patients with polycystic ovary syndrome. *Frontiers in Nutrition*, 9, 1018674. https://doi.org/10.3389/fnut.2022.1018674

12 'low-carb Mediterranean diet helped to restore menstrual cycles and hormone levels in overweight PCOS patients, and was significantly more effective than a low-fat diet': Mei, S., Ding, J., Wang, K., Ni, Z., & Yu, J. (2022). Mediterranean Diet Combined With a Low-Carbohydrate Dietary Pattern in the Treatment of Overweight Polycystic Ovary Syndrome Patients. *Frontiers in Nutrition*, 9, 876620. https://doi.org/10.3389/fnut.2022.876620

12 'polyphenols (plant compounds) and adequate fibre in our diet also helps to maintain and feed the different colonies of bacteria that live in our gut': Zhou, P., Feng, P., Liao, B., Fu, L., Shan, H., Cao, C., Luo, R., Peng, T., Liu, F., & Li, R. (2024). Role of polyphenols in remodeling the host gut microbiota in polycystic ovary syndrome. *Journal of Ovarian Research*, 17(1), 69. https://doi.org/10.1186/s13048-024-01354-y

12 'Those with PCOS may have an imbalance of bacteria in the gut microbiome, driving chronic inflammation': Singh, S. et al. (2023). Polycystic Ovary Syndrome.

13 'turmeric': Chien YJ, Chang CY, Wu MY, Chen CH, Horng YS, Wu HC. Effects of Curcumin on Glycemic Control and Lipid Profile in Polycystic Ovary Syndrome: Systematic Review with Meta-Analysis and Trial Sequential Analysis. *Nutrients* 2021;13:684. https://doi.org/10.3390/nu13020684

13 'ginger': Huang, F. Y., Deng, T., Meng, L. X., & Ma, X. L. (2019). Dietary ginger as a traditional therapy for blood sugar control in patients with type 2 diabetes mellitus: A systematic review and meta-analysis. *Medicine*, 98(13), e15054. https://doi.org/10.1097/MD.0000000000015054

13 'cinnamon': Dou, L., Zheng, Y., Li, L., Gui, X., Chen, Y., Yu, M., & Guo, Y. (2018). The effect of cinnamon on polycystic ovary syndrome in a mouse model. *Reproductive Biology and Endocrinology: RB&E*, 16(1), 99. https://doi.org/10.1186/s12958-018-0418-y

13 'Green tea': Maleki, V., Taheri, E., Varshosaz, P., Tabrizi, F. P. F., Moludi, J., Jafari-Vayghan, H., Shadnoush, M., Jabbari, S. H. Y., Seifoleslami, M., & Alizadeh, M. (2021). A comprehensive insight into effects of green tea extract in polycystic ovary syndrome: a systematic review. *Reproductive Biology and Endocrinology: RB&E*, 19(1), 147. https://doi.org/10.1186/s12958-021-00831-z

13 'spearmint tea': Grant P. (2010). Spearmint herbal tea has significant anti-androgen effects in polycystic ovarian syndrome. A randomized controlled trial. *Phytotherapy Research: PTR*, 24(2), 186–188. https://doi.org/10.1002/ptr.2900

13 'nettle tea': Grant, P., & Ramasamy, S. (2012). An update on plant derived anti-androgens. *International Journal of Endocrinology and Metabolism*, 10(2), 497–502. https://doi.org/10.5812/ijem.3644

14 'Refined carbohydrates': Barrea, L., Marzullo, P., Muscogiuri, G., Di Somma, C., Scacchi, M., Orio, F., Aimaretti, G., Colao, A., & Savastano, S. (2018). Source and amount of carbohydrate in the diet and inflammation in women with polycystic ovary syndrome. *Nutrition Research Reviews*, 31(2), 291–301. https://doi.org/10.1017/S0954422418000136

15 'exercise can be another tool […] to aid insulin sensitivity': Shele, G., Genkil, J., & Speelman,

217

D. (2020). A Systematic Review of the Effects of Exercise on Hormones in Women with Polycystic Ovary Syndrome. *Journal of Functional Morphology and Kinesiology*, 5(2), 35. https://doi.org/10.3390/jfmk5020035

15 '**Resistance training and building muscle mass in particular can help to reduce insulin resistance that may be driving hyperandrogenism (excess facial and body hair), and can help to increase metabolic rate**': Wright, P. J., Corbett, C. F., Pinto, B. M., Dawson, R. M., & Wirth, M. (2021). Resistance Training as Therapeutic Management in Women with PCOS: What is the Evidence?. *International Journal of Exercise Science*, 14(3), 840–854. https://doi.org/10.70252/NEEX8658

16 '**Zinc**': Jamilian, M., Foroozanfard, F., Bahmani, F., Talaee, R., Monavari, M., & Asemi, Z. (2016). Effects of Zinc Supplementation on Endocrine Outcomes in Women with Polycystic Ovary Syndrome: a Randomized, Double-Blind, Placebo-Controlled Trial. *Biological Trace Element Research*, 170(2), 271–278. https://doi.org/10.1007/s12011-015-0480-7

16 '**Vitamin D**': Łagowska K, Bajerska J, Jamka M. The role of vitamin D oral supplementation in insulin resistance in women with polycystic ovary syndrome: a systematic review and meta-analysis of randomized controlled trials. *Nutrients* 2018;10:1637. https://doi.org/10.3390/nu10111637

16 '**Inositol**': Sharon P, M., P, M., Manivannan, A., Thangaraj, P., & B M, L. (2024). The Effectiveness of Myo-Inositol in Women With Polycystic Ovary Syndrome: A Prospective Clinical Study.

Cureus, 16(2), e53951. https://doi.org/10.7759/cureus.53951

16 '**Turmeric or curcumin**': Abdelazeem B, Abbas KS, Shehata J, Baral N, Banour S, Hassan M. The effects of curcumin as dietary supplement for patients with polycystic ovary syndrome: An updated systematic review and meta-analysis of randomized clinical trials. *Phytother Res* 2022;36:22-32. https://doi.org/10.1002/ptr.7274

16 '**Omega-3 or fish oil**': Yang, K., Zeng, L., Bao, T., & Ge, J. (2018). Effectiveness of Omega-3 fatty acid for polycystic ovary syndrome: a systematic review and meta-analysis. *Reproductive Biology and Endocrinology: RB&E*, 16(1), 27. https://doi.org/10.1186/s12958-018-0346-x

16 '**N-acetyl cysteine (NAC)**': Nemati, M., Nemati, S., Taheri, A. M., & Heidari, B. (2017). Comparison of metformin and N-acetyl cysteine, as an adjuvant to clomiphene citrate, in clomiphene-resistant women with polycystic ovary syndrome. *Journal of Gynecology Obstetrics and Human Reproduction*, 46(7), 579–585. https://doi.org/10.1016/j.jogoh.2017.07.004

16 '**CoQ10**': Gutierrez-Mariscal, F. M., de la Cruz-Ares, S., Torres-Peña, J. D., Alcalá-Diaz, J. F., Yubero-Serrano, E. M., & López-Miranda, J. (2021). Coenzyme Q10 and Cardiovascular Diseases. *Antioxidants* (Basel, Switzerland), 10(6), 906. https://doi.org/10.3390/antiox10060906

16 '**Vitamin E**': Heidari, H., Hajhashemy, Z., & Saneei, P. (2022). A meta-analysis of effects of vitamin E

supplementation alone and in combination with omega-3 or magnesium on polycystic ovary syndrome. *Scientific Reports*, 12(1), 19927. https://doi.org/10.1038/s41598-022-24467-0

16 '**Magnesium**': Simental-Mendía, L. E., Sahebkar, A., Rodríguez-Morán, M., & Guerrero-Romero, F. (2016). A systematic review and meta-analysis of randomized controlled trials on the effects of magnesium supplementation on insulin sensitivity and glucose control. *Pharmacological Research*, 111, 272–282. https://doi.org/10.1016/j.phrs.2016.06.019

17 '**oral contraceptive pill**': https://www.nhs.uk/conditions/polycystic-ovary-syndrome-pcos/treatment/

Glossary of UK/US Terms

UK	US
aubergine	eggplant
beetroot	beet
bicarbonate of soda	baking soda
broad bean	fava bean
cake tin	cake pan
caster sugar	superfine sugar
chickpea	garbanzo beans
clingfilm	plastic wrap
coriander	cilantro
courgette	zucchini
desiccated coconut	dried unsweetened shredded coconut
frying pan	skillet
grill	broiler
kitchen paper	paper towels
minced	ground
plain flour	all-purpose flour
prawn	shrimp
rocket	arugula
sieve	strainer
spring onion	scallion
vanilla pod	vanilla bean

Index

INDEX

Acknowledgements

Thank you to my family, friends and to Ben for your constant support.

To the women I have the privilege to support each day – thank you for your trust, your commitment, and the opportunity to be part of your health journeys. Your experiences shaped the direction of this work and contribute to improving care for all women with PCOS.

About the Author

Megan Hallett is a registered nutritional therapist (mBANT, rCNHC) who specializes in women's health. Since being diagnosed with PCOS at the age of 18, the focus of her practice has been supporting hormonal health through nutrition.

www.meganhallett.com
Instagram.com/meganhallettnutrition

Picture Credits